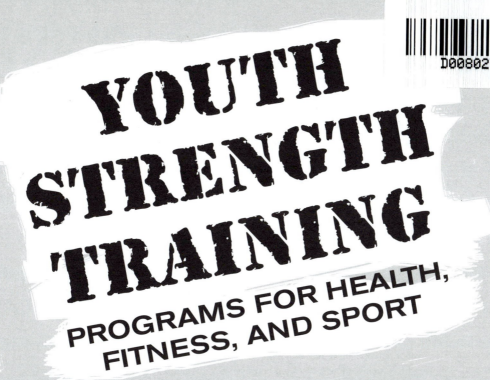

YOUTH STRENGTH TRAINING

PROGRAMS FOR HEALTH, FITNESS, AND SPORT

Avery D. Faigenbaum, EdD, CSCS
The College of New Jersey

Wayne L. Westcott, PhD, CSCS
South Shore YMCA, Quincy, Massachusetts

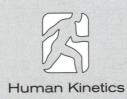

Human Kinetics

Library of Congress Cataloging-in-Publication Data

Faigenbaum, Avery D., 1961-
    Youth strength training : programs for health, fitness, and sport /
Avery D. Faigenbaum, Wayne L. Westcott. -- 2nd ed.
        p. cm. -- (Strength & power for young athletes)
    Rev. ed. of: Strength & power for young athletes, c2000.
    Includes bibliographical references and index.
    ISBN-13: 978-0-7360-6792-8 (soft cover)
    ISBN-10: 0-7360-6792-2 (soft cover)
    1. Exercise for children. 2. Physical fitness for children. I.
Westcott, Wayne L., 1949- II. Faigenbaum, Avery D., 1961- Strength &
power for young athletes. III. Title.
    RJ133.F35 2009
    613.7'042--dc22

                                                    2008049096

ISBN-10: 0-7360-6792-2 (print)   ISBN-10: 0-7360-8761-3 (Adobe PDF)
ISBN-13: 978-0-7360-6792-8 (print)   ISBN-13: 978-0-7360-8761-2 (Adobe PDF)

Copyright © 2009, 2000 by Avery D. Faigenbaum and Wayne L. Westcott

This book is a revised edition of *Strength & Power for Young Athletes,* published in 2000 by Human Kinetics.

Acquisitions Editor: Scott Wikgren; **Developmental Editor:** Melissa Feld; **Assistant Editor:** Rachel Brito; **Copyeditor:** Jan Feeney; **Indexer:** Craig Brown; **Permission Manager:** Dalene Reeder; **Graphic Designer:** Nancy Rasmus; **Graphic Artist:** Denise Lowry; **Cover Designer:** Keith Blomberg; **Photographer (cover):** Neil Bernstein; **Photographer (interior):** Neil Bernstein, except where otherwise noted. Photos on pages 1, 16, 170, 183, and 209 © Human Kinetics. Photo on page 167 © MM Productions/Corbis; **Visual Production Assistant:** Joyce Brumfield; **Photo Production Manager:** Jason Allen; **Art Manager:** Kelly Hendren; **Associate Art Manager:** Alan L. Wilborn; **Illustrators:** Andrew Recher, page 18, and Alan L. Wilborn; **Printer:** Versa Press

We thank the South Shore YMCA in Quincy, Massachusetts, for assistance in providing the location for the photo shoot for this book.

Printed in the United States of America   10 9 8 7 6 5 4 3 2 1

The paper in this book is certified under a sustainable forestry program.

Human Kinetics
Web site: www.HumanKinetics.com

United States: Human Kinetics, P.O. Box 5076, Champaign, IL 61825-5076
800-747-4457
e-mail: humank@hkusa.com

Canada: Human Kinetics, 475 Devonshire Road Unit 100, Windsor, ON N8Y 2L5
800-465-7301 (in Canada only)
e-mail: info@hkcanada.com

Europe: Human Kinetics, 107 Bradford Road, Stanningley, Leeds LS28 6AT, United Kingdom
+44 (0) 113 255 5665
e-mail: hk@hkeurope.com

Australia: Human Kinetics, 57A Price Avenue, Lower Mitcham, South Australia 5062
08 8372 0999
e-mail: info@hkaustralia.com

New Zealand: Human Kinetics, Division of Sports Distributors NZ Ltd., P.O. Box 300 226 Albany, North Shore City, Auckland
0064 9 448 1207
e-mail: info@humankinetics.co.nz

It is with great appreciation
that we dedicate this book to the hundreds of boys and girls
who have participated so enthusiastically in our strength training programs,
to their most accommodating parents
who genuinely appreciated the importance
of developing a strong musculoskeletal system at a young age,
and to all the fitness professionals and physical education teachers
with whom we have worked to help youth understand
the value of regular strength training as a lifestyle choice.

CONTENTS

PART III PROGRAM DESIGN

PART IV LONG-TERM PLANNING AND NUTRITIONAL SUPPORT

FOREWORD

I am pleased to introduce Avery Faigenbaum and Wayne Westcott's book *Youth Strength Training: Programs for Health, Fitness, and Sport.* Their first book on this topic *(Strength & Power for Young Athletes),* published in 2000, was groundbreaking because it introduced the principles as well as the practical aspects of developing safe and effective strength-training programs for children and adolescents.

Using the 2000 book as its foundation, this new edition presents a large scope of new information on youth strength-training programs. This reflects the growing interest and research in this area as well as the experience of strength and fitness professionals in the training of young athletes. Although much has been learned in the intervening years, it is still apparent that teachers and coaches need to follow the age-appropriate strength-training guidelines that Drs. Faigenbaum and Westcott present in this well-researched text.

The International Olympic Committee's Consensus Statement on Training the Elite Child Athlete, which was published in March of 2008 in the *Clinical Journal of Sports Medicine,* is a summary of the available scientific information regarding training elite child athletes. This consensus statement notes the need for further research in this area because there is increased emphasis on systematic training and participation in organized sports by children and adolescents. Despite this worldwide trend and concerns about the safety

and efficacy of sport conditioning for this age group, the authors have provided sensible and specific exercise guidelines for youth strength training based on their two decades of research on this topic.

Youth Strength Training: Programs for Health, Fitness, and Sport contains the most current scientifically based information on strength and power training for young athletes. This new edition is even more detailed and specific in its recommendations for developing enjoyable and effective strength-training programs for youth of all abilities. Although the focus of this book is on the training of young athletes, the principles embodied here can be used for any child or adolescent as part of a general conditioning and fitness program.

I highly recommend this book for anyone involved in the training of children and adolescents. It is a valuable resource that you will turn to frequently for assistance in designing youth strength-training programs.

Lyle J. Micheli, MD
O'Donnell family professor
of orthopaedic sports medicine
Children's Hospital Boston,
Harvard Medical School
Director of Division of Sports Medicine
Children's Hospital Boston
Past president of American College
of Sports Medicine

ACKNOWLEDGMENTS

It is a great privilege to acknowledge the many gifted individuals who so generously gave their time and talents in helping us write this book. We are most grateful for the professional leadership at Human Kinetics. We especially appreciate the editorial expertise of Melissa Feld and the superb photography skills of Neil Bernstein. We thank Gabrielle Burgess, Gary Burgess, Andrew DeLacey, Lisa DeLacey, and Jennifer DeLacey for demonstrating correct exercise technique for the photos. We are also indebted to the parents of the models, Gary and Diane Burgess and Brian and Lynn DeLacey, for their unwavering support of our youth strength-training programs and extraordinary assistance during the photo sessions.

We are particularly grateful to registered dietitian Debra Wein for her nutrition advice and Rita LaRosa-Loud for her innovative leadership in our youth strength-training classes. We appreciate the support from Patrick Mediate, Jim McFarland, and Tracy Radler, who allowed us to use their weight rooms and gymnasiums as our research labs. We especially thank Ralph Yohe and the directors of the South Shore YMCA for our state-of-the-art youth strength-training facility.

We thank the many student interns who have provided outstanding exercise instruction and research assistance in our youth strength-training programs. Finally, we sincerely appreciate the support of Dr. Lyle Micheli and his sports medicine staff at Boston Children's Hospital for our youth strength-training programs over the past 20 years.

INTRODUCTION

Our first edition of *Youth Strength Training: Programs for Health, Fitness, and Sport* presented the physiological and psychological benefits associated with regular resistance exercise in boys and girls 7 to 15 years of age. In the nine years since the publication of the first edition, we have completed more research studies, compiled more data, taught more unfit children, worked with more youth athletes, and presented more pertinent information in the area of muscular conditioning programs for young people. One of the most compelling reasons for youth strength training is the development of a strong musculoskeletal system that can withstand the rigors of sport participation as well as ward off the degenerative effects of the aging process. We now know that the time to build bone is during the preteen through teenage years and that children who regularly perform resistance exercise increase bone mineral density several times as fast as those who do not strength train.

Another health benefit of youth strength training is improved body composition, which is particularly important in light of the present epidemic of childhood obesity. One out of three children is challenged by excessive body fat, and these boys and girls are poorly suited for both endurance-type exercise and fast-paced athletic activities, which they typically avoid at all costs. Fortunately, they generally enjoy performing resistance exercise, most likely because they compare more favorably with their lighter peers and they find the training effects highly reinforcing (that is, they look better, feel better, and function better).

When it comes to sport participation, few things rival resistance exercise for reducing risk of injury and enhancing athletic performance. Tiger Woods is a perfect example of this, as are the members of the women's cross-country team at Notre Dame High School in Hingham, Massachusetts. Over a four-year period, these female athletes combined their running workouts with sensible strength training under our supervision. The results were remarkable. The superbly conditioned Notre Dame teams (15 varsity runners and 15 junior varsity runners) won four consecutive New England cross-country championships and had only one injury during the entire four years of competition. Contrary to the misconceptions that strength training increases the potential for injury and decreases endurance performance, the facts are that properly executed strength exercise enhances running economy and reduces the risk of muscle overuse and imbalance problems.

Although our first book focused on the safety and effectiveness of youth strength training, we now have new research for designing more efficient, enjoyable, productive, and practical programs of strength exercise for young people of various ages and abilities. In addition to our studies on workout frequency, exercise sets and repetitions, and related training components, we have examined other factors that affect program design for both sport conditioning and general fitness for essentially all boys and girls. In fact, the primary focus of this book is to help physical education teachers, coaches, and parents provide the best program of resistance exercise for youth to develop a functional level of strength fitness and a desirable body composition. Our research indicates that improving these physical characteristics is reinforcing to all young people regardless of size, shape, or athletic abilities.

In addition to producing more effective and efficient strength-training programs, our new research has led to the development of more productive protocols for warming up and cooling down, more acceptable procedures for enhancing joint flexibility, and more innovative means of incorporating resistance exercises into physical education classes, sport practice sessions, and exercise facilities at YMCAs, fitness centers, and home settings. Recently, we implemented a strength-training program with medicine balls at a local high school. The results were so impressive and the students enjoyed the program so much that this program is now part of a statewide physical education curriculum in 1st through 12th grade. This school is now ranked as one of the top schools in the state for physical fitness assessment scores.

We have also expanded our information in the areas of nutrition and recovery to maximize the beneficial effects of strength exercise for all children as well as to minimize the risks of overtraining in young athletes. Emphasis is placed on a broad base of balanced muscle development for every boy and girl, and the secondary objective is performing more specific strength-training protocols for youth who participate in various sports and recreational activities. Once they achieve an acceptable level of overall muscle conditioning, youth sport participants will find more comprehensive strength-training programs for numerous athletic activities within the general categories of power sports, jumping sports, striking sports, and endurance sports.

Teachers, coaches, and parents who incorporate our latest muscular conditioning programs should see high rates of strength development and few overuse injuries among their young trainees. Because children are not miniature adults, we do not simply offer a watered-down version of adult strength-training programs. In fact, children of various ages and developmental levels respond best to specifically designed protocols of resistance exercise. We therefore present age-specific strength-training programs for students in elementary school (7 to 10 years), middle school (11 to 14 years), and high school (15 to 18 years). Because children experience varying rates of physiological development, we provide guidelines for individualizing the general

exercise protocols within each age group. We also present a specially designed section on athletic conditioning for a variety of sports. The information is comprehensive, and the organization is easy to understand and apply.

Based on our combined 50 years of experience in teaching youth strength-training classes and coaching all kinds of athletes, as well as our research on instructional techniques, we devote an entire chapter to the art and science of educating and motivating young people to properly perform resistance exercise. Toward this end, we place a strong emphasis on exercise selection and performance, as evidenced by the clear illustrations and precise descriptions of more than 100 resistance exercises using weight stack machines, free weights, medicine balls, elastic bands, and body-weight resistance.

We believe that proper exercise technique is the most critical concern in presenting and instructing youth strength-training programs. Although the number of exercises, sets, and repetitions youth perform are important aspects of workout design, *how* they perform each exercise, set, and repetition has even more impact on the safety and success of their training sessions. And that is the underlying theme throughout this book: training for the right purpose and purposely training in the right manner to maximize musculoskeletal development and minimize risk of injury in children and young athletes. If you are interested in childhood obesity, youth fitness, or sport conditioning, then *Youth Strength Training: Programs for Health, Fitness, and Sport* is the definitive text for implementing efficient and research-based exercise programs for your children, physical education classes, and sport teams.

PART I
FITNESS FUNDAMENTALS

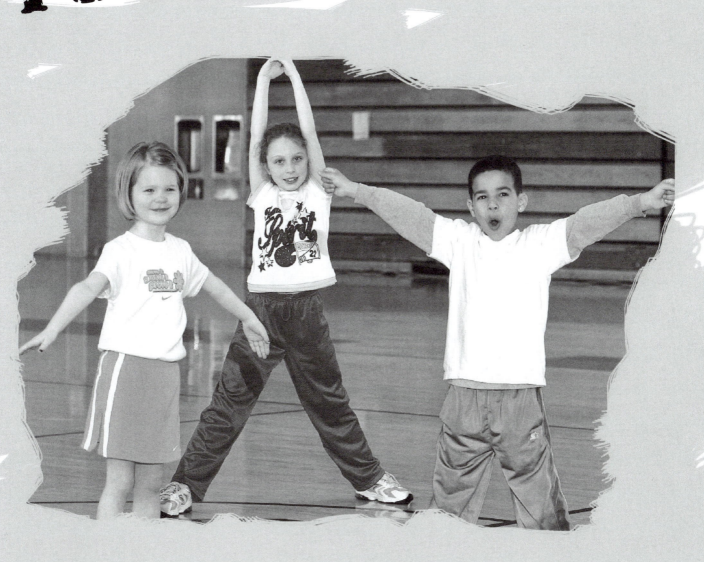

FITNESS FUNDAMEN

READY TO TRAIN

Children and adolescents need to participate regularly (i.e., most days of the week) in 60 minutes or more of moderate to vigorous physical activity that is developmentally appropriate, enjoyable, and varied. While aerobic activities such as swimming and bicycling are generally recommended for youth, scientific evidence and clinical impressions indicate that strength training can offer unique benefits for boys and girls provided that age-appropriate training guidelines are followed. With proper guidance and instruction, regular participation in a youth strength-training program can have favorable effects on musculoskeletal health, body composition, cardiovascular risk factors, fitness performance, and psychological well-being. Furthermore, a stronger musculoskeletal system will enable youth to perform life's daily activities with more energy and vigor and may increase young athletes' resistance to sport-related injuries.

During our youth, physical activity did not involve a conscious decision to engage in planned exercise; rather, it was what we did on a regular basis before, during, and after school. Regular physical activities that involved running, jumping, lifting, balancing, throwing, and kicking not only kept our bodies healthy, fit, and strong, but were important for our cognitive, motor skill, and social development. But today, youth seem to spend more time in front of televisions and computer screens than at the playground. The bottom line is that a sedentary lifestyle during childhood and adolescence may increase the risk of developing some chronic diseases such as heart disease, diabetes, and osteoporosis later in life. Thus, it is even more important to encourage youth to be physically active on most days of the week as part of play, recreation, physical education, sports, and transportation.

Physical education teachers, youth coaches, and fitness instructors need to create opportunities for boys and girls of all abilities to be physically active. While organized sport programs certainly have their place, participation in physical activity should not begin with competitive sport; it should evolve out of preparatory conditioning that includes strength training. That is, children should participate in a variety of physical activities that enhance their motor performance skills and improve their musculoskeletal strength in order to better prepare them for the demands of daily sport practice and competition. Focusing entirely on specific sport skills at an early age not only limits the ability of children to succeed at tasks outside a narrow physical spectrum but also discriminates against children whose motor skills develop at a slower pace.

Our youth fitness pyramid (figure 1.1) illustrates the importance of first preparing the musculoskeletal systems of youth for the demands of more vigorous physical activity and sport competition through regular participation in general exercise and what we call FUNdamental fitness conditioning. Unlike other physical activity pyramids that focus on early sport participation, the youth fitness pyramid highlights the importance of FUNdamental fitness conditioning (which includes strength, power, aerobic, flexibility, and agility exercises) before sport-specific training and competition. Enjoyable youth programs that develop both health- and skill-related components of physical fitness will be more likely to spark a lifelong interest in physical activity and sport.

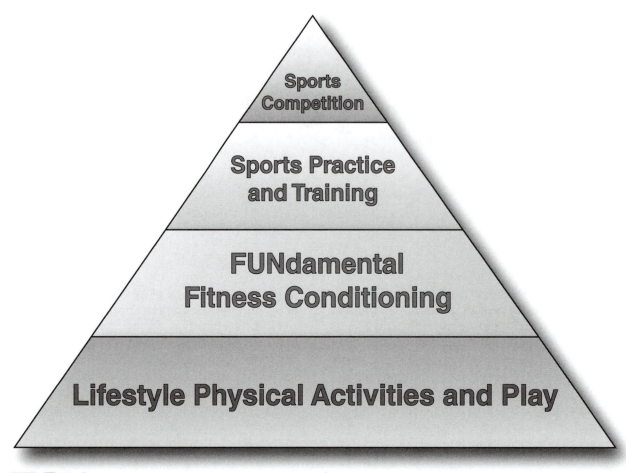

Figure 1.1   Youth fitness pyramid.

You've probably heard that children should not train with weights because it doesn't work, places too much stress on growing muscles, or is dangerous. Categorically, all of these reasons are misconceptions. As you are undoubtedly aware, strength-building exercise can be beneficial to growing boys and girls. However, because children are not miniature adults, you must progress cautiously when training young people. Over the past several years, research has clearly demonstrated that strength exercise is a safe, effective, and efficient means for conditioning young muscles, as long as certain safety precautions are in place. Fortunately, all the boys and girls in our program have increased their muscular strength, and not one has had an exercise-related injury. This is most likely due to the careful supervision that we provide to all our strength-training participants.

Others also recommend strength training for young people. Several medical and fitness organizations, including the American Academy of Pediatrics, the American College of Sports Medicine, the American Council on Exercise, the British Association for Sport and Exercise Science, the Canadian Society for Exercise Physiology, the National Association for Sport and Physical Education, and the National Strength and Conditioning Association, have published guidelines for youth strength training. That's a pretty impressive list of supporters for youth strength training.

Furthermore, the American Alliance for Health, Physical Education, Recreation and Dance developed a comprehensive school-based program called Physical Best, which enhances young people's ability to perform physical activities that require aerobic fitness, joint flexibility, and muscular strength. By incorporating components of health-related physical fitness into the elementary and secondary school curricula, school-age youth will gain the knowledge and confidence they need in order to be physically active adults.

In addition, strength training during childhood and adolescence may provide the foundation for dramatic gains in muscle strength during adulthood. Thus, the key issue is not only appreciating the potential health-related benefits of strength training for youth but understanding how to provide children and adolescents with the skills, knowledge, attitudes, and behaviors that lead to a lifetime of muscle-enhancing physical activity.

What's more, regular participation in a youth strength-training program can have a favorable impact on skill-related fitness components, including power, speed, balance, coordination, agility, and reaction time. Although a high degree of skill-related fitness is not a prerequisite for a lifetime of physical activity, confidence and competence in the ability to perform skills that require balance, coordination, and power can indeed contribute to a person's health and fitness throughout both youth and adult years. For example, since strength training can enhance muscular strength and muscular power, which are required for success in all sports including tennis, basketball, and track, it is likely that youth who strength train will perform better than those who do not strength train.

Moreover, as sport performance improves, the activity will become more enjoyable and therefore participants will be more likely to stick with it. Thus, unlike other modes of exercise training that typically isolate fitness components, strength training provides physical education teachers with an opportunity to integrate health- and skill-related fitness components into a comprehensive physical education program in which all children can feel challenged while they enhance both health- and skill-related fitness abilities (see table 1.1). While it is important not to overemphasize skill development, we believe the best approach is to teach all students to recognize the value of both health- and skill-related fitness components.

> Strength training provides physical education teachers with an opportunity to integrate health- and skill-related fitness components into a comprehensive physical education program in which all children can feel challenged while they enhance both health- and skill-related fitness abilities.

Table 1.1 Components of Fitness

Health-related fitness	Skill-related fitness
Aerobic fitness	Agility
Muscular strength and endurance	Coordination
Flexibility	Reaction time
Body composition	Balance
	Speed
	Power

Strength Training Versus Weightlifting, Powerlifting, and Bodybuilding

Strength training is different from weightlifting, powerlifting, and bodybuilding. By definition, strength training is a planned and structured means of exercising with appropriate resistance that a participant gradually progresses as the musculoskeletal system becomes stronger. Children and adolescents can perform strength training with a variety of equipment, such as weight machines, free weights (barbells and dumbbells), elastic bands, medicine balls, or body weight alone. Properly designed and supervised youth strength-training programs should involve enjoyable activities in which every participant gains strength and experiences success in a safe and supportive exercise environment.

Weightlifting and powerlifting are competitive sports in which participants typically train with moderate and heavy weights in order to maximize gains in muscle strength and muscle power. In the sport of weightlifting, athletes perform the clean and jerk and snatch exercises; in the sport of powerlifting, athletes perform the squat, bench press, and deadlift exercises. Bodybuilding is a competitive sport in which the goal is to maximize gains in muscle size, symmetry, and definition. Although many of the exercises that weightlifters, powerlifters, and bodybuilders perform are described in this book, we focus on the principles and programs for designing progressive youth strength-training programs that are fundamental for all school-age youth. Model programs for young competitive lifters are available through professional organizations such as USA Weightlifting. Other terms commonly used in designing youth strength-training programs are defined in table 1.2.

> Properly designed and supervised youth strength-training programs should involve enjoyable activities in which every participant gains strength and experiences success in a safe and supportive exercise environment.

FUNdamental Fitness

There are two broad categories of youth, and both need strength training to develop and enhance fundamental locomotor (e.g., running), nonlocomotor (e.g., lifting), and manipulative (i.e., throwing) skills that are the components of most games and sports. The larger category consists of those boys and girls who engage in little physical activity on a regular basis. Unlike children in earlier generations, they don't do many physical chores, don't play backyard sports, don't have many physical education classes, and don't engage in much vigorous activity. Sadly, increasing urbanization has resulted in a lack of safe play areas, and many boys and girls spend most of their free time in passive pursuits such

Table 1.2 Definition of Common Terms

Term	Definition
Agility	The ability to quickly decelerate, change direction, and accelerate again.
Balance	The maintenance or control of a body position.
Coordination	The ability of various muscles to work together to produce a specific movement.
Local muscular endurance	The ability to perform repeated repetitions with a submaximal, or moderate, load.
Muscular fitness	The ability to perform physical activities that require muscular strength, muscular power, or local muscular endurance.
Plyometrics	A type of power training that consists of jumping, hopping, and throwing activities.
Power	The rate of performing work. The product of force and velocity.
Reaction	A response to a stimulus.
Repetition	One complete movement of an exercise.
Repetition maximum	The maximum number of repetitions that can be performed with a given resistance.
Set	A group of repetitions performed continuously without resting.
Speed	The ability to achieve high velocity.
Strength	The maximal amount of force a muscle or muscle group can generate.
Strength training	Also called resistance training. A specialized method of conditioning that involves the progressive use of a wide variety of resistive loads and a variety of training modalities designed to enhance muscular fitness.

as watching television, playing video games, or surfing the Internet. This lack of regular physical activity has contributed to the unabated increase in the prevalence of obesity among children and adolescents. Over the past three decades, the prevalence of childhood obesity has more than doubled for adolescents and has more than tripled for children. And the likelihood that an obese child will become an obese adult is both real and alarming.

Since obese youth may lack the motor skills and confidence to be physically active, they may actually perceive physical activity to be discomforting and embarrassing. Thus, these youth desperately need strength training to condition their muscles, tendons, ligaments, and bones because a fundamental level of musculoskeletal fitness is essential for youth to experience and enjoy a physically active lifestyle. Although strength training is not often associated with a high caloric expenditure, obese youth are less willing and often unable to participate in prolonged periods of moderate to vigorous aerobic exercise. Not only does excess body weight hinder the performance of weight-bearing physical activity such as jogging, but the risk of musculoskeletal overuse injuries is also a concern.

Strength training provides obese youth with a positive activity that enables them to enjoy purposeful exercise, experience personal improvement, and train cooperatively with friends in a supportive setting and exciting atmosphere. Observations from our youth strength-training centers suggest most obese children and adolescents find strength training activities enjoyable because this type of exercise is not aerobically taxing and provides an opportunity for all youth, regardless of body size, to experience success and feel good about their performance. Furthermore, since obese youth tend to use the heaviest weight loads, they typically receive unsolicited feedback from their peers who are often impressed with the amount of weight they can lift. The first step in encouraging obese children and adolescents to exercise may be to increase their confidence in their ability to be physically active, which in turn may lead to an increase in regular physical activity, a noticeable improvement in muscle strength, and exposure to a form of exercise that can be carried into adulthood. Our review of the literature, which was published in the *President's Council on Physical Fitness and Sports Research Digest,* clearly indicates that participation in a supervised program of strength exercise can make a world of difference in a child's life.

The other category of young people consists of the sport participants. These are the kids who play soccer; do age-group swimming; take dance, gymnastics, and skating lessons; and participate in other organized sport activities. Although they get plenty of physical exercise, they also need a general program of strength training to ensure balanced muscle development and lower their risk for overuse injuries. Basically, children should have good overall strength before engaging in competitive sports that can place excessive stress on an unconditioned musculoskeletal system. An overemphasis on sport-specific skills typically provides too little stimulus for some major muscles and too much stress on other major muscles; therefore, injury, failure, and frustration are the likely results.

Muscles, Bones, and Connective Tissue

The concept of fundamental fitness revolves around developing a strong and fit musculoskeletal system. The musculoskeletal system consists of the muscles, tendons, ligaments, and bones that enable us to move and perform physical activities. A strong musculoskeletal system prepares children for all types of physical activity and reduces the risk of sport-related injuries. Few things have as much of a positive effect on a young person's life as a well-conditioned musculoskeletal system.

You might have heard that children do not have sufficient levels of the muscle-building hormone testosterone to gain strength apart from normal growth and maturation. This is a false assumption. Although preadolescents and females of all ages have too little natural testosterone to develop large muscles, they can certainly increase their muscle strength. Boys and girls in research studies typically improved their muscle strength by 30 to 50 percent in only two months of training. This is possible because strength development is associated with a variety of neuromuscular factors and does not solely depend on hormone levels.

> A strong musculoskeletal system prepares children for all types of physical activity and reduces the risk of sport-related injuries. Few things have as much positive impact on a young person's life as a well-conditioned musculoskeletal system.

Another misconception concerns growth retardation in children who train with weights. Nothing could be further from the truth. There has never been a report of stunted growth or reduced bone formation related to strength training. While bone mass is strongly influenced by genetics, progressive strength exercise makes bones stronger and more resistant to injury. Because most bone mass is accrued during childhood and adolescence, this is the ideal time to enhance musculoskeletal strength and structure through properly designed resistance-training programs. In addition to the direct effect of strength exercise on bone, strength training can increase bone mass indirectly by increasing muscle strength, which in turn can increase the stress placed on bone. Hence, training-induced gains in muscle strength allow for even greater forces to be placed on bone where the strengthened muscles attach. This may be particularly beneficial for young girls in reducing their risk of osteoporosis later in life.

Program Assessment

When properly administered, fitness assessments can be used for evaluating specific strengths and weaknesses, developing personalized programs, tracking progress, and motivating participants. Standardized testing procedures for assessing physical fitness have been developed, and normative data are available for most health-related assessments. However, when evaluating youth, it is important to avoid the pass–fail mentality because this approach may actually discourage unfit or overweight boys and girls from participating in physical education class or other physical activity programs. In an attempt to create an environment in which students enjoy the fitness assessment and feel good about participating,

we refer to the assessment as a challenge rather than a test. As such, every student is rewarded for participating, and youth who try their best but do not have the ability to perform a minimal number of repetitions receive a + instead of a 0.

In a clinical or research setting, children typically perform a variety of physical tests that assess muscular fitness. The most common strength tests determine the repetition maximum (RM), which is the maximum amount of weight that can be lifted for a specific number of repetitions. For example, a 1RM is the most weight that can be lifted once but not twice on an exercise, and a 10RM is the most weight that can be lifted for 10 but not 11 repetitions. Normally, clinicians or researchers will determine the RM on two or three multijoint exercises. With close supervision, qualified instruction, adequate warm-up, and an appropriate progression of loads, RM strength testing can be a safe and effective method for assessing muscular strength and evaluating training-induced gains in muscular fitness in youth. However, RM strength testing is labor intensive and requires a lot of time, since several trials with adequate rest between trails are required to accurately determine the maximal weight that can be lifted for a predetermined number of repetitions. An example of a testing protocol used for determining a 1RM is outlined in the sidebar.

> When properly administered, fitness assessments can be used for evaluating specific strengths and weaknesses, developing personalized programs, tracking progress, and motivating participants.

Other types of fitness assessments are available for physical education teachers and youth coaches who work with large groups of children and adolescents. These assessments are relatively easy to administer and provide valid and reliable information on selected measures of health and fitness. Furthermore, since the most worthwhile youth programs inspire children and teenagers to develop lifelong healthy habits, these fitness assessments provide students with an opportunity to demonstrate what they can do now that they could not do before. The Fitnessgram is

PROCEDURE FOR ONE-REPETITION MAXIMUM STRENGTH TEST

1. Perform 5 minutes of dynamic warm-up activities.
2. Start with 5 repetitions using 50 percent of the estimated 1RM.
3. After a 1-minute rest, perform 3 repetitions with 70 percent of the predicted 1RM.
4. After a 2-minute rest, perform 1 repetition with the estimated 1RM.
5. If the lift was successful, increase the load and perform a second 1RM trial after a 2-minute rest. The increments in weight should be dependent on the effort required to complete the lift and should become progressively smaller as the weight approaches the 1RM.

Repeat step 5 until the child is unable to complete 1 repetition with proper form. Typically, 3 to 5 trials are needed in order to determine a 1RM. Failure is defined as a trial falling short of the full range of motion on 2 attempts separated by at least 2 minutes.

an example of a comprehensive health-related assessment of individual fitness that can help students incorporate physical activity into their lives. Along with personal responsibility and goal setting, the Fitnessgram can help all school-age youth achieve and maintain a realistic level of fitness that is associated with good health. For example, by setting performance benchmarks that are in the so-called healthy fitness zone, students can set realistic goals and monitor their progress in attaining them.

In addition to the activities in the standard Fitnessgram, physical education teachers and youth coaches can incorporate skill-related fitness assessments into their fitness challenges. Since skill-related assessments that involve jumping, sprinting, and throwing require power, speed, and agility, performance on these activities can be used in evaluating the effectiveness of strength-training programs and assessing aspiring young athletes' readiness for sport training and competition. Our research indicates that performance on the long jump and vertical jump is related to 1RM strength and therefore may be useful for assessing muscular fitness in school-age youth. Not only are skill-related assessments inexpensive and easy to administer, but the incorporation of skill-related assessments into the fitness challenge may provide boys and girls in the low range of health-related fitness with an additional opportunity to feel good about participating in fitness activities.

Although no universally accepted youth fitness challenge exists, the Fitnessgram along with

selected skill-related fitness activities provides the best overall assessment for school-age youth who participate in a strength-training program. Since training-induced adaptations are, in part, specific to the type of muscle actions performed during strength exercises, the fitness challenge should include both health- and skill-related activities in order to provide a more comprehensive fitness assessment. You can administer the fitness challenge all at once, or you can select various components that match the concepts you're covering in your practices or class. For example, when you're teaching concepts of upper-body muscular conditioning, relating the push-up and medicine ball assessments to the concepts discussed will enhance motivation and provide a sense of purpose for assessing muscular fitness.

Fitnessgram Assessments

The Fitnessgram assesses muscular strength and muscular endurance of the upper body and the trunk region. The curl-up and trunk extensor exercises assess strength and endurance of the trunk muscles, which are important for good posture and the maintenance of health of the lower back health. Upper-body strength and endurance are typically assessed with the 90-degree push-up, although a pull-up, modified pull-up, or flexed arm hang are alternatives. The Fitnessgram uses criterion-referenced standards in evaluating fitness performance. That is, performance in the so-called healthy fitness zone, or HFZ, represents a level of fitness that offers some degree of protection against disease, whereas youth who perform in the needs improvement zone should be encouraged to participate in activities that will develop those specific areas. Additional information about interpreting Fitnessgram results appears in the *Fitnessgram Test Administration Manual* and posted at www.fitnessgram.net. Descriptions of Fitnessgram assessments for muscular strength and muscular endurance appear in the following paragraphs.

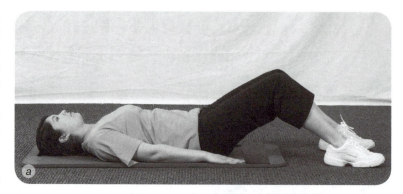

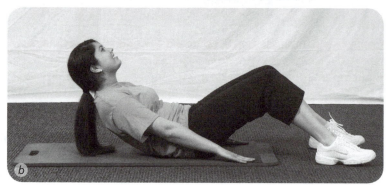

Figure 1.2 Curl-up.

• **Curl-up.** Participant lies face-up on a mat with knees bent at 140 degrees, feet flat, and arms straight and parallel to the trunk with palms on the mat (see figure 1.2*a*). For children under 10 years of age, place a 3-inch (7.6 cm) measuring strip next to the fingertips. For children 10 years of age and older, use a 4.5-inch (11 cm) strip next to the fingertips. Participant curls up slowly, sliding fingers across the strip until fingertips reach the other side (see figure 1.2*b*), then returns to starting position. Cadence is about 1 curl-up every 3 seconds. Participant continues without pausing until he or she can no longer continue or has completed 75 curl-ups.

• **Trunk lift.** Participant lies facedown on a mat with hands under thighs (see figure 1.3*a*). Place a marker on the floor in line with the child's

eyes. Participant lifts the upper body off the floor to a maximum height of 12 inches (30 cm) in a slow and controlled manner (see figure 1.3*b*). During the movement, the participant's eyes should remain focused on the marker. Participant holds this position as the distance from the floor to his or her chin is measured, then participant returns to starting position. The ruler should be placed 1 inch in front of the participant's chin. Record the best of two trials in inches; 12 inches (30 cm) is the maximum score.

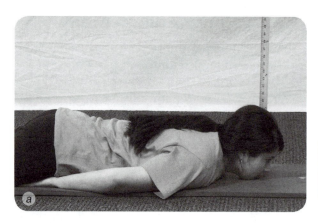

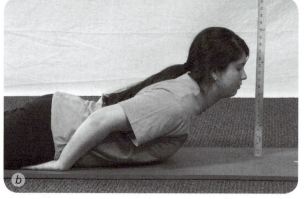

Figure 1.3 Trunk lift.

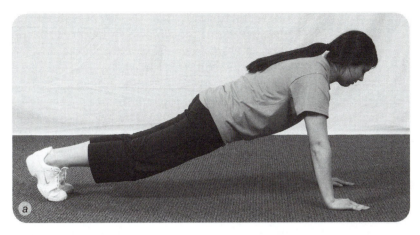

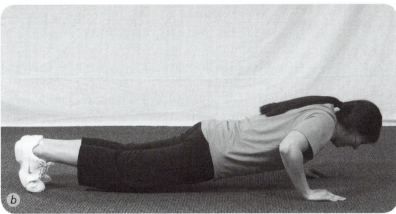

Figure 1.4 Push-up.

• **90-degree push-up.** This exercise is used in assessing strength and endurance in the chest, shoulder, and arm muscles. Participant assumes a facedown position on a mat with hands placed slightly wider than shoulders and legs straight. Participant pushes up off the mat until arms are straight (see figure 1.4a). While keeping the back in a straight line, participant lowers the body until both elbows are at 90 degrees and the upper arms are parallel to the floor (see figure 1.4b). Participant returns to the starting position and repeats as many times as possible. Cadence is about 1 push-up every 3 seconds.

Skill-Related Fitness Assessments

The following skill-related fitness activities can also be used in assessing individual performance and evaluating the effectiveness of your strength-training program. As with any fitness assessment, physical education teachers or youth coaches should demonstrate the proper performance of

each skill, provide an opportunity for each participant to practice a few repetitions, and offer guidance and instruction when necessary. Since skill-related assessments are relatively quick and easy to administer, they should be performed before Fitnessgram activities. In our classes and after-school programs, we use the vertical jump, long jump, and seated medicine ball toss in assessing muscular power. In addition to using pretraining and posttraining scores for evaluating performance, you can use norms for selected skill-related fitness tests available at Exercise Prescription on the Net (www. exrx.net).

• **Vertical jump.** Participant stands with the dominant shoulder about 6 inches (15 cm) from a wall with both feet flat on the floor. Participant reaches as high as possible with the dominant hand and marks the height reached on a wall-mounted board or yardstick (see figure 1.5a). Participant lowers the hand and then, without a stutter step, quickly bends the knees and hips and jumps upward (see figure 1.5b). Participant touches the board or yardstick as high as possible with the dominant hand. The vertical jump is calculated by subtracting the standing reach height from the maximal jump height. The best of three trials should be recorded to the nearest 0.5 inch.

• **Long jump.** Participant stands with the toes just behind the starting line on a long jump mat (see figure 1.6a). He or she quickly bends the knees and hips and then jumps forward as far as possible (see figure 1.6b). The long jump is the distance from the starting line to the back edge of the rearmost heel. The best of three trials should be recorded to the nearest 0.5 inch.

• **Seated medicine ball toss.** Participant sits on the floor while holding a medicine ball (2 to 4 lb, or 1 to 2 kg, for children and 6 lb, or 3 kg, for teenagers) with both hands against the chest (see figure 1.7a). Participant tosses

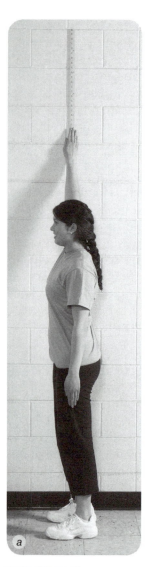 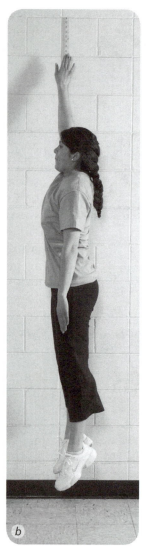

Figure 1.5 Vertical jump.

the ball as far as possible with both hands at an approximate angle of 45 degrees (see figure 1.7*b*). Participant releases the ball when it is above the level of the head. The distance from the starting line (near the toes) to the near edge of the mark on the floor made by the ball is measured. The best of three trials should be recorded to the nearest inch.

Getting Ready

Under normal circumstances, it is not mandatory for apparently healthy children to have a medical examination before doing strength exercise. Of course, a physician should screen

any child with known or suspected health problems, including illness or injury, before he or she participates in a strength-training program. The training environment should be safe and free of any potential hazards, and exercises should be performed on a nonskid surface. Accessories such as lifting belts and gloves are not essential, but all youth should wear proper-fitting footwear with nonslip soles.

Although there is no minimum age requirement for doing strength exercise, children should exhibit adequate emotional maturity in order to understand and follow directions before participating in a strength-training program. All participants should have a positive attitude toward the strength-training program. You should not force children to continue who do not look forward to their strength-training sessions. As a point of reference, many 7- and 8-year-old boys and girls have successfully completed our youth strength-training programs. In fact, in over 15 years of after-school strength-training classes, the average dropout rate was less than 5 percent.

> A physician should screen any child with known or suspected health problems, including illness or injury, before he or she participates in a strength-training program.

Because of age, size, and maturational differences, it is essential to address each child's needs and abilities when designing the strength-training program. Since physiological functions are more closely related to biological age than chronological age, you should personalize the exercise protocol and training procedures as much as possible. Because an early-maturing youth has a strength advantage over a late-maturing child, emphasize individual progress and avoid weight-load comparisons. For example, a class of sixth-grade students can have a height difference as great as 9 inches (23 cm) and a weight difference that exceeds 50 pounds (23 kg). Furthermore, a 12-year-old girl might be taller and stronger than a 12-year-old boy. These differences are due to variations in the timing

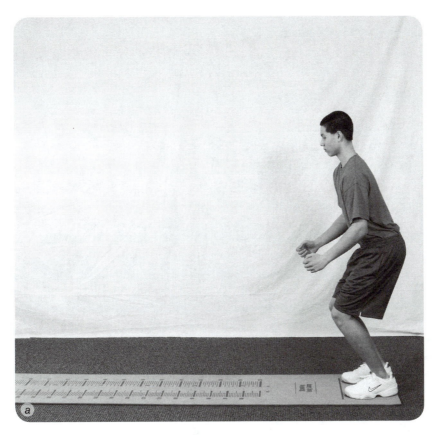

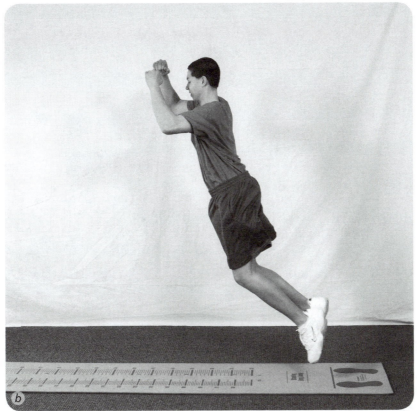

Figure 1.6 Long jump.

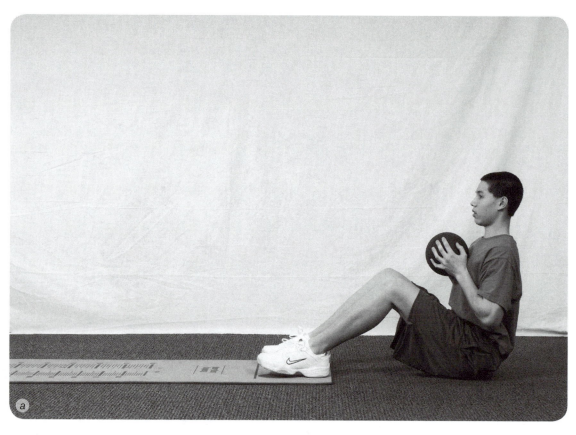

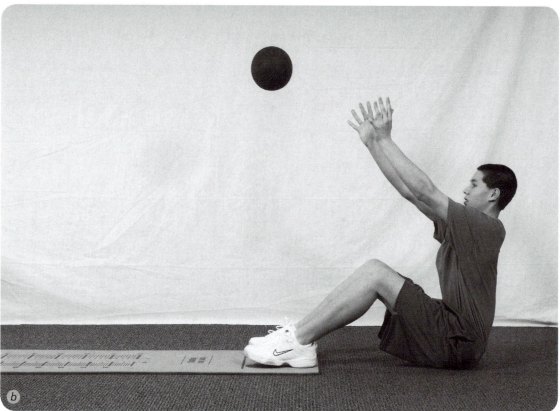

Figure 1.7 Seated medicine ball toss.

and magnitude of growth during puberty. We advise that you address the reasons for program differences, because most children appreciate an ability-based approach to training.

Sensitivity to individual differences and abilities is especially important when teaching children and adolescents. An early-maturing 12-year-old girl may be ready to participate in an advanced conditioning program, whereas a late-maturing 14-year-old boy might not be ready for the demands of a structured strength-training program. Teachers and coaches need to think about children's desire to strength train as well as their ability to understand and follow directions. In addition, a child's training age (the length of time a child has been strength training) should also be considered because the magnitude of gains in strength is affected by the amount of adaptation that has already taken place. For example, a 16-year-old with 2 years of strength-training experience (i.e., training age of 2 years) may not achieve the same strength gains in a given period as a 12-year-old with no strength-training experience (training age of 0).

Perhaps the most important consideration in youth strength-training programs is that children are not merely miniature adults. Standard adult workout protocols may not be best for young people. For example, during the first few weeks of strength training, children respond better to high-repetition training (13 to 15 repetitions) than to low-repetition training (6 to 8). You must also understand that strength programs practiced by collegiate and professional athletes are unacceptable for boys and girls with immature bodies. Remember that children are less developed physically and psychologically, and they participate in strength training for different reasons than adult athletes do. Basically, young strength trainers are motivated by learning new skills, making new friends, and having fun while exercising. Attempting to sell strength training to children on the basis that it can improve their

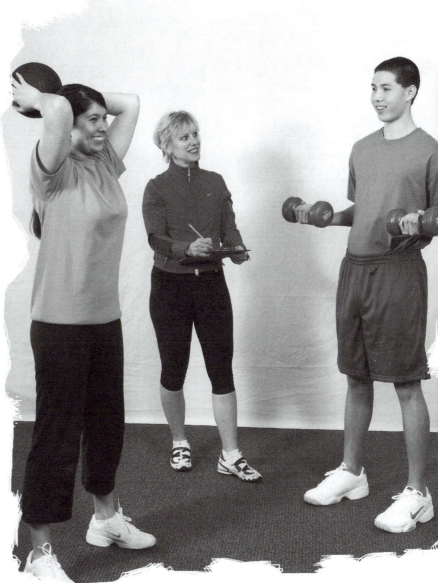

Boys and girls can benefit from sensible strength training.

quality of life is a losing proposition. The focus of youth activity programs should be on positive experiences instead of stressful competition in which most children fail.

Acknowledging that there are some inherent risks in all physical endeavors, a properly designed and supervised strength-training program is a safe, purposeful, and productive activity for young people. In fact, strength training provides the opportunity for progressive challenges and recurrent successes while building both physical prowess and self-confidence.

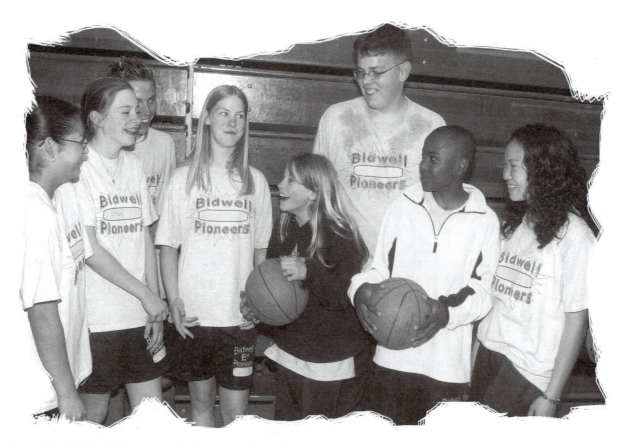

Recognize individual differences when working with youth.

Summary

Medical and fitness organizations now promote strength training for children and adolescents, provided that they follow appropriate training guidelines. In addition to increasing the strength of muscles, bones, and connective tissue, regular participation in a strength-training program may better prepare young athletes for sport participation and reduce the number and severity of sport-related injuries. With competent instruction, health- and skill-related fitness assessments, meaningful feedback on performance, and effective use of practice time, boys and girls can learn the skills for successful and enjoyable participation in strength-training activities.

2

PROGRAM PRESCRIPTIONS

With appropriate guidance, youth can have fun while conditioning their muscles and developing a positive attitude about strength-training activities. The program we suggest allows both children and adolescents the opportunity to work in a safe and stimulating environment through individually prescribed exercise methods.

You can strive for a health-enhancing program by introducing the many benefits of strength training and emphasizing the importance of proper form and technique. Place a high priority on education and motivation, which encourage boys and girls to take a positive and sensible approach to their strength-training program. We post pictures of boys and girls performing strength-training exercises next to the equipment in order to remind participants of proper exercise technique. We also promote our program on posters, create Web sites about youth strength and conditioning, and develop educational handouts about our program for parents and participants. Of course, having competent instruction and attentive supervision is most helpful, and a low teacher–student ratio is important.

Our basic advice for successful youth strength training is to design personalized programs that accommodate each child's physical abilities. Intense exercise sessions with short rest periods certainly have their place, but most children find such programs too demanding and discouraging. We believe it is better to underestimate participants' physical abilities and progress gradually to more difficult workouts and heavier weight loads than to do too much too soon and encounter setbacks or injuries. In other words, when working with weight trainers of any age, it is always better to undertrain than to overtrain.

We have regular and relevant conversations with the children, listening carefully to their concerns as well as giving them plenty of feedback and positive reinforcement. On the other hand, we consistently and fairly enforce the training rules, foremost of which is the performance of each exercise with proper technique. Our primary objectives are to help each child master his or her training system, understand the potential benefits of strength training, record workout information, monitor personal progress, and spark a lifelong interest in physical activity.

Since children who continue to improve their health and fitness are more likely to adhere to the exercise program, key factors in the design of any youth strength-training program are the inclusion of specific exercises that will strengthen the major muscle groups and the manipulation of program variables that will keep the strength-training program fresh and effective. All of the major muscle groups are illustrated in figure 2.1. We post daily workouts on a bulletin board and regularly modify training programs to optimize gains and reduce boredom. While we encourage all participants to try their best, we realize that the importance of creating an enjoyable exercise experience for all participants should not be overlooked.

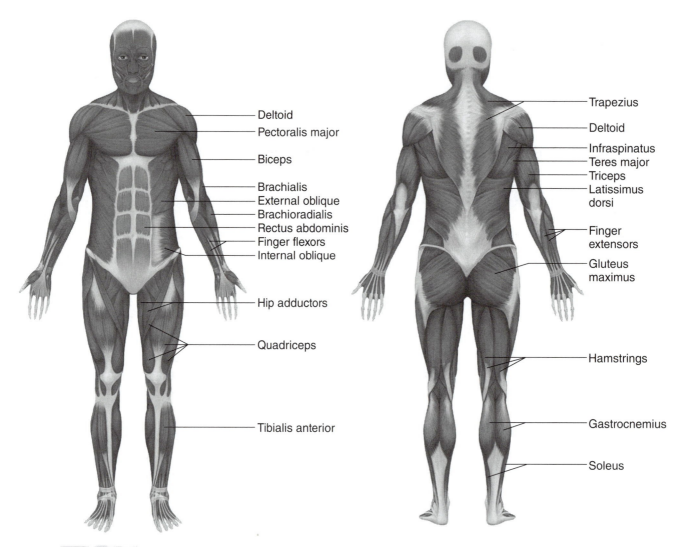

Figure 2.1 Major muscle groups of the human body.

We accept no form of horseplay in the exercise area. While our warm-up and cool-down components involve activities such as aerobic dance, locomotor games, calisthenics, and relays, we do everything with a purpose. If a child feels weak or fatigued, we adjust the training session accordingly. We make every effort to help the children feel competent, confident, and comfortable in the exercise environment.

Keep in mind that a safe exercise setting must be spacious, uncluttered, well ventilated, and well lighted. All training equipment should be in good working order and properly sized for the participants. While most adolescents are too tall for child-sized weight machines, they can use adult-sized weight machines with an extra pad or board if needed to ensure proper fit. Most children are too small for adult-sized machines,

so child-sized weight machines, medicine balls, and free weights such as barbells and dumbbells are viable alternatives for small boys and girls. Be sure to provide adequate space around each exercise station and keep the floor clear of barbells, dumbbells, weight plates, and other materials. We insist that the youth dress appropriately for exercise, with supportive athletic shoes and clothing that permit freedom of movement.

Training Guidelines

Because of variations in maturation, training age, and stress tolerance, youth strength-training programs need to be prescribed and progressed carefully. In addition, cautionary measures such as qualified supervision and health screening need to be considered when children and adolescents want to participate in a strength-training program. Several prominent exercise and medical associations have developed specific guidelines for safe, sensible, and successful youth strength-training programs. These strength-training guidelines combined with our years of experience in working with children and adolescents in the weight room provide the foundation for our youth strength-training recommendations.

> Because of variations in maturation, training age, and stress tolerance, youth strength-training programs need to be prescribed and progressed carefully.

The program variables in designing a youth program are choice and order of exercise, training intensity (resistance and repetitions), training sets, rest interval between sets and exercises, repetition velocity, and training frequency.

Choice and Order of Exercise

With respect to the choice of strength equipment, we believe that sound training techniques and teaching methods are more important than the mode of exercise. For example, we have experienced excellent training effects from youth programs using free weights (barbells and dumbbells), medicine balls and weight machines (pushing and pulling exercises), and child-sized machines (weight stacks and plate loaded). We have also used elastic bands and body-weight exercises. All have proven safe and productive when children practice the prescribed training procedures and are taught how to perform each exercise correctly.

Although every mode of training has its advantages and disadvantages, the type of exercise equipment used in training should be consistent with the needs, goals, and abilities of each participant. Additionally, the equipment should be safe, free of defects, cost effective, and located in an uncrowded area free of obstructions with adequate lighting and ventilation. The information in this book will enable youth to attain excellent strength development on all types of exercise equipment.

Although a limitless number of exercises can be used for enhancing strength, we suggest beginning with basic exercises for the major muscle groups, such as the leg press, leg curl, chest press, seated row, shoulder press, biceps curl, and triceps press-down. We also emphasize midsection exercises for the typically underdeveloped lower-back and abdominal muscles. Trunk curls and trunk extensions performed with body weight or with a medicine ball work well for this purpose and thus reduce the injury risk to this vulnerable area of the body.

The choice of exercises not only should be appropriate for a child's exercise experience but should also promote muscle balance across joints and between opposing muscle groups (e.g., quadriceps and hamstrings). In our youth strength-training programs we start with simple exercises and gradually progress to more challenging exercises that require more coordination and skill to perform correctly. In general, youth should perform about 8 to 12 strength exercises during each training session. Table 2.1 presents standard free-weight and machine exercises available on youth-sized equipment that address the major muscle groups and are appropriate for beginners.

Since most youth will perform total-body workouts consisting of multiple exercises that stress all the major muscle groups, exercises of the larger muscle groups should be performed before exercises of smaller muscle groups, and multijoint exercises should be performed before single-joint exercises. It is also helpful to perform power-enhancing exercises earlier in the workout when participants are less fatigued. For example, if a child is learning how to perform a cone jump or a weightlifting movement such as the power clean, this type of exercise should be performed early in the workout so the movement can be practiced correctly without undue fatigue.

Training Intensity

The most important variable in the design of a strength-training program is the training intensity. To maximize gains in muscle strength, youth must first learn how to perform each exercise correctly with a relatively light weight or wooden dowel and then learn how to add the appropriate amount of resistance. Individual effort combined with a well-designed strength-training program will ultimately determine the adaptations that take place.

Table 2.1   Standard Free-Weight and Machine Exercises for the Major Muscle Groups

	Free-weight exercises	Machine exercises*
Front thigh (quadriceps)	Dumbbell squat Dumbbell lunge Dumbbell step-up	Leg extension Leg press
Rear thigh (hamstrings)	Dumbbell squat Dumbbell lunge Dumbbell step-up	Leg curl Leg press
Inner thigh (hip adductors)	Dumbbell side lunge	Hip adduction
Outer thigh (hip abductors)	Dumbbell side lunge	Hip abduction
Lower leg (gastrocnemius and soleus)	Dumbbell heel raise	Heel raise
Chest (pectoralis major)	Dumbbell bench press	Chest press
Upper back (latissimus dorsi)	Dumbbell one-arm row Dumbbell pullover	Seated row Pullover Front pull-down
Shoulders (deltoids)	Dumbbell lateral raise	Overhead press
Front arms (biceps)	Dumbbell biceps curl Dumbbell incline biceps curl	Biceps curl
Rear arms (triceps)	Dumbbell triceps kickback Dumbbell triceps overhead extension	Triceps extension
Lower-back extension (erector spinae)	Prone back raise	Lower-back extension
Abdominals (rectus abdominis)	Trunk curl	Abdominal curl

*Weight machines are available in adult and child sizes.

Since the act of strength training itself does not result in health and fitness benefits unless the training stimulus exceeds a minimal threshold, it has been recommended that youth perform 6 to 15 repetitions of each exercise with proper technique and that the last few repetitions should result in temporary muscle fatigue. However, our research studies have enabled us to make a few refinements that enhance both the efficiency and efficacy of training. For example, we have com-pared preadolescent strength gains achieved from fewer repetitions (6 to 8) using heavy weight loads with gains attained from more repetitions (13 to 15) using moderate weight loads. Unlike the findings for adult strength training, our findings indicate that preadolescent boys and girls do better with higher repetitions and moderate weight loads during the first two months of training. When prescribing a strength-training program for youth, the best method may be to first establish the repetition range (e.g., 10 to 15) and then by trial and error determine the weight that can be lifted with proper form for the prescribed repetition range. This approach not only allows for positive changes in muscular performance but also provides an opportunity for necessary adjustments to be made within the appropriate repetition range.

Since it can take several sessions to determine an appropriate strength-training intensity for inexperienced weight trainers, we developed a child-specific rating scale of perceived exertion to aid in the prescription of strength exercise. Our newly developed scale is called the perceived exertion for children scale and contains verbal expressions along a numerical response range from 0 to 10 and five pictorial descriptors that represent a child at various levels of exertion while lifting weights (figure 2.2). After the completion of the last repetition, children are asked to rate their level of exertion using the numbers on the scale to describe how their muscles felt during the exercise set. We have found that an effort rating of 6 or 7 is consistent with a training intensity of approximately 75 percent maximum. Although the relationship between repetitions and selected percentages of maximum strength might vary between muscle groups, most youth can typically perform about 10 repetitions at an intensity of 75 percent maximum. We use this information along with our assessment of each participant's physical exertion and training experience to aid in the prescription of the training intensity.

Training Sets

It is reasonable to begin strength training with one set on a variety of exercises and then gradually progress to multiple sets depending on program goals and class time. Our studies suggest that beginners who perform one high-effort set of each exercise experience excellent strength gains. Therefore, single-set resistance training is an efficient means for increasing muscle strength in young boys and girls during the first few weeks of strength training.

After the initial adaptation period, performing two or three sets per exercise may lead to even greater strength development over time, especially if done progressively. Our participants have attained their greatest strength gains using the DeLorme-Watkins training protocol, which requires a low-, moderate-, and high-effort set of each exercise. That is, the participant performs the first set with a light resistance for 10 repetitions, the second set with a moderate resistance for 10 repetitions, and the third set with a heavy resistance for 10 to 15 repetitions. When he or she can complete 15 repetitions, the resistance is increased slightly in all three sets. While this combination of sets and repetitions has proven to be most effective for youth, remember that not all exercises need to be performed for the same number of sets and repetitions. In most cases, it is reasonable to begin strength training with one or two sets and then progress to three sets on selected multijoint movements depending on individual goals and time available for training.

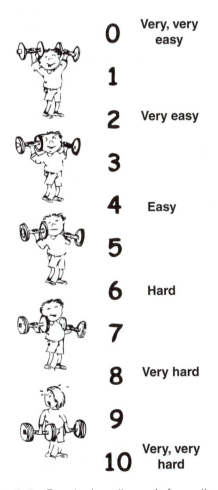

Figure 2.2 Perceived exertion scale for youth.

Rest Interval Between Sets and Exercises

The amount of recovery between sets and exercises is an important but sometimes overlooked training variable. The length of rest between sets and exercises influences energy recovery and the training adaptations that take place. Although rest periods of 2 to 3 minutes are typically recommended for adults who strength train, recent findings have shown that children and teenagers are able to recover from physical exertion faster than adults. Thus, a rest period between sets and exercises of 1 minute for children and 1 to 2 minutes for teens is appropriate for most youth strength-training programs. Although even shorter rest intervals may be appropriate for fitness circuit training, longer rest intervals are not recommended because youth have shorter attention spans than adults; therefore, prolonged rest periods between sets and exercises might result in boredom and horseplay.

We recommend shorter rest periods between sets and exercises to keep youth focused. If participants are completing multiple sets and you notice that performance begins to wane after the first set, alter the training program and lengthen the rest interval. In any case, participants should have enough recovery time between sets to perform each exercise correctly at the desired intensity.

Repetition Velocity

The velocity, or cadence at which an exercise is performed, can affect the adaptations to a training program. Although young people are prone to doing things quickly, we insist on exercise control achieved through moderate-speed lifting and lowering movements on traditional strength-building exercises such as the chest press and back squat. We generally require about 4 to 6 seconds for each repetition: 2 to 3 seconds for the concentric, or lifting, phase of the exercise and 2 to 3 seconds for the eccentric, or lowering, phase of the movement. We believe that controlled speeds maximize strength development and minimize the risk of injury. Because fast movement on weight machines involves momentum, it might reduce the effect of the exercise and the safety of the training. However, it is important to realize that different various velocities may be used depending on the choice of exercise and

training goals. For example, the leg press exercise should always be performed at a controlled movement speed to enhance muscle strength and minimize the risk of injury. Conversely, exercises such as the power clean, 90-degree jump, and some medicine ball exercises such as the chest pass are controlled exercises that should be performed at a high velocity. Emphasize that the coordination and exercise technique required for learning these movements correctly may require an unloaded barbell or lightweight medicine ball.

Training Frequency

Our youth strength-training studies have shown similar results from two or three exercise sessions per week. On the one hand, most boys and girls like the strength-training program and are willing to exercise three days per week. On the other hand, two weekly workouts may make more sense for young people who are involved in additional physical activities such as dance, gymnastics, swimming, tennis, or team sports.

While training once per week may maintain training-induced gains in strength, our research has shown that strength training only once per week is suboptimal for developing strength in youth. After several weeks of progressive strength training, children who exercised once per week achieved 67 percent of the gains as those who trained twice per week. Thus, we suggest a training frequency of two or three times per week on nonconsecutive days in order to optimize training adaptations while allowing for adequate recovery between training sessions (48 to 72 hours).

Program Considerations

Youth should genuinely appreciate the benefits and risks associated with strength training, and teachers and coaches should have a solid understanding of strength-training principles. If you adhere to the following considerations, youth strength training has the potential to be a pleasurable and valuable experience.

1. Participants must have the emotional maturity to accept and follow instruction.
2. There must be adequate supervision by teachers and coaches who are knowledgeable about strength training and who

genuinely appreciate the uniqueness of childhood and adolescence.

3. Strength training should be part of a comprehensive program to increase both health- and skill-related fitness.

4. Participants should precede strength training with dynamic warm-up activities and end each workout with cool-down stretching.

5. The program should emphasize concentric and eccentric muscle actions.

6. Participants should perform all exercises through a full range of motion.

Although we recognize the value of traditional stretch-and-hold exercises, we incorporate static stretching exercises into the cool-down of our physical education classes and youth sport programs rather than during the warm-up portion. Although warm-up protocols that include static stretching have become standard practice, over the past few years long-held beliefs about the potential benefits of warm-up static stretching have been questioned. There has been a growing interest in warm-up procedures that involve the performance of dynamic hops, skips, jumps, and lunges that elevate body temperature, enhance the excitability of muscle fibers, improve kinesthetic awareness, and maximize active ranges of motion. Since muscles are actually turned on during dynamic warm-up activities, they will be better prepared for strength-training activities. Specific recommendations for designing dynamic warm-up protocols are outlined in chapter 8.

> Although warm-up protocols that include static stretching have become standard practice, over the past few years long-held beliefs about the potential benefits of warm-up static stretching have been questioned.

Play Education

Both art and science are involved in well-designed youth strength-training programs. While the science is in understanding the principles of strength training, the art is in understand-

ing how to design a safe, effective, and enjoyable strength-training program for participants with varying needs, goals, and abilities. Thus, the goal of youth strength training should not be limited to increasing muscle strength but should also include teaching children about their bodies, promoting an interest in fitness, and having fun. The concept of fun can be defined in various ways, but we like to define fun as a balance between skill and challenge. If children don't have the skills to perform an exercise, strength training won't be fun. And if an exercise is too challenging for a child, that won't be fun either. But if a child has the knowledge, skills, and confidence to perform an exercise and feels somewhat challenged by the task at hand, that's when strength training becomes fun.

> While the science is in understanding the principles of strength training, the art is in understanding how to design a safe, effective, and enjoyable strength-training program for participants with varying needs, goals, and abilities.

We put as much effort into promoting positive attitudes as we put into promoting the physical aspects of the strength-training program. We promote gradual improvement and continually remind the students that it takes time to develop strength and master new skills. We also stress training consistency and reward the children for regular participation. We keep track of attendance on a large poster board that we display in our youth fitness center. We ask children who regularly come to class to assist with exercise demonstrations, and teenagers who have graduated from our program sometimes return to provide encouragement and instruction. We often treat the class to heart-healthy snacks, and at the end of each program all participants receive a certificate of completion that recognizes personal improvement and achievement of realistic goals. Throughout the program we take the time to acknowledge birthdays, graduations, and other special events.

To avoid a winners-and-losers atmosphere in the weight room, we emphasize intrinsic factors

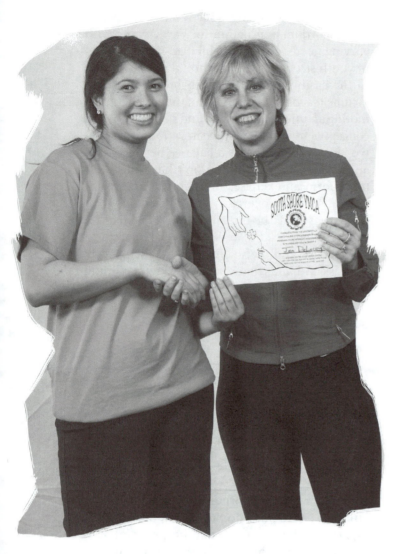

Students like to receive certificates of completion for their training.

and individual achievement without comparing weight loads or performance abilities. For example, we use personal workout logs so the children record their own training efforts and focus on individual improvement. We encourage each participant to ask questions, and we interact as much as possible with every boy and girl. We sometimes stop an exercise to correct technique or reduce the resistance if the child is not performing it properly. However, we do our best to make all recommendations in a positive and friendly manner, working together to attain our training objectives.

Summary

The prescribed strength-training program for children and adolescents should include a variety of exercises that address the major muscle groups of the body. Children and adolescents can safely use various types of equipment, including weight machines, free weights, medicine balls, and resistance bands, provided that participants have qualified supervision and they understand the importance of proper exercise technique. Teachers and coaches need to address individual needs and concerns and should fairly enforce training rules for the safety of all participants. Don't overlook the importance of having fun and developing a positive attitude toward strength-training activities. With appropriate guidance and supervision, children and adolescents can learn to embrace self-improvement and feel good about their accomplishments.

3

EXERCISE TECHNIQUE AND TRAINING PROCEDURES

Strength training can be a safe way to condition the musculoskeletal system if the program is followed appropriately and within guidelines. Despite preconceived notions, research studies indicate that youth who participate in supervised strength-training programs have a lower risk of injury than youth who participate in other sports and activities. In fact, it seems that the forces children place on their musculoskeletal systems when participating in strength training are likely to be less in duration and magnitude of exposure than what they would generate by participating in soccer, football, or gymnastics.

Although adults and children who strength train may have similar goals, the focus of youth strength-training programs should be on intrinsic factors such as skill improvement, personal successes, and having fun. We place a high value on participation and positively reinforce children who actively participate in the workouts. Adults need to realize that the slogan "No pain, no gain" does not apply when working with boys and girls, most of whom have never experienced strength exercise before. Most adults and children enjoy physical activity if it is developmentally appropriate. That is, the activity needs to be consistent with each participant's age, ability, interests, and experience.

Yet we are troubled by the increasing number of participants who drop out of youth fitness programs because the training was too intense, too time consuming, or simply not fun. Parents, teachers, and coaches need to understand the uniqueness of children and the importance of adhering to safety concerns. The focus of our program is not on the amount of weight that children can lift but on developing proper form and technique for a variety of strength-building exercises. This is particularly important when teaching beginners multijoint free-weight exercises that require more skill, balance, and coordination. Our goal is to teach children how to strength train properly so that they can continue this exercise for a lifetime.

To ensure safety in your youth strength-training program, you need to take the following steps:

- Parents must complete a health history questionnaire on each child. If there is evidence of a preexisting medical condition, such as diabetes, the parents must obtain a physician's approval before the child begins the program.

- Instructors must make sure the exercise area is adequately ventilated and free of clutter.

- Children should wear comfortable attire that does not restrict movement patterns and athletic footwear that provides good traction and prevents slipping.

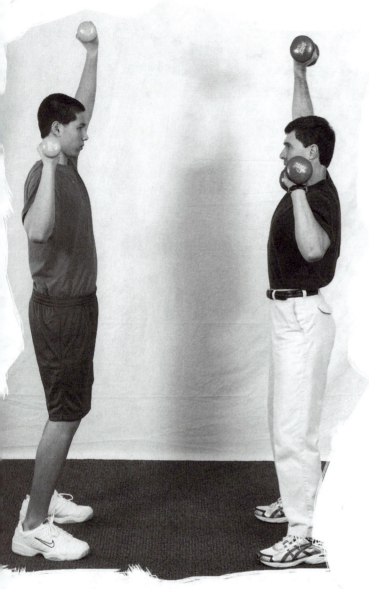

Demonstrate proper lifting technique for each exercise.

- When strength training, children must not wear necklaces of any type, including those that hold keys.
- Children should not chew gum during class.
- Children should drink water before, during, and after class.
- Instructors must begin strength training with light weights to allow for appropriate adjustments in training loads.
- Children should focus on proper exercise technique rather than the amount of weight they lift.
- Children should learn correct breathing

techniques and should not hold their breath when lifting.
- Instructors who are knowledgeable in youth fitness and strength training must supervise every class.

Understanding Children

Knowledgeable adults who understand and appreciate the physical and psychological characteristics of children are the most important factor in children's strength-training experience. Unlike adults, children are still growing and are therefore more prone to certain types of injury. For example, children who do not follow age-appropriate strength-training guidelines may damage the growth cartilage located at the end of long bones, near the tendon insertions, and on the joint surfaces. Although injuries to the growth cartilage have been reported in young weight trainers, these injuries typically happened when untrained children attempted to press near-maximum weights overhead in an unsupervised environment. Fortunately, this type of injury has not been reported in any youth strength-training research study that incorporated an appropriate progression of training loads and close supervision. To minimize the chance of injury to the growth cartilage, children should always follow proper and progressive training procedures. For example, all participants should learn how to perform free-weight exercises with a light load, a wooden dowel, or a piece of PVC piping and use proper form and technique. Once participants have established movement competency, they can progress to an aluminum barbell with plastic training plates.

Damage to the growth cartilage can also occur if children repeatedly participate in sports and recreational activities without giving their bodies a chance to recover. The problem is that repetitive stress to the growing area of the bone results in microtraumas, which need time to heal and recover. Without adequate recovery, the microtraumas eventually result in what is commonly known as an overuse injury. Although strength training can reduce the incidence of overuse injuries in youth sport participants, it is

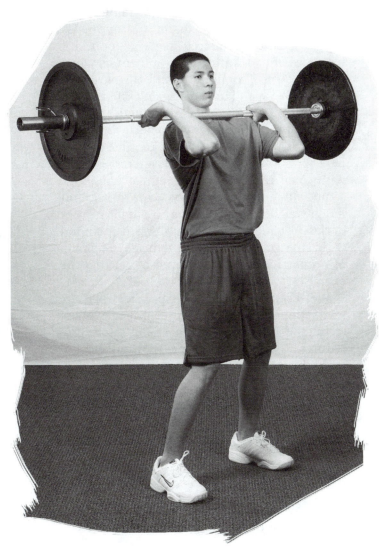

Following proper and progressing training procedures will allow youth to progress to an aluminum barbell and plastic training plates.

believe that you should design strength training into a year-round conditioning program that changes periodically. During this time children can improve their overall fitness levels, and you can identify and correct any specific needs, such as muscle imbalances. By enhancing muscular fitness before sport participation, you help young athletes improve their general athletic skills and reduce their risk of injury. You are also likely to increase their willingness to participate in physical activities. Furthermore, a stronger musculoskeletal system will allow them to use their sport-specific skills at a higher level of play. In some cases, children may need to decrease the time they spend practicing sport-specific skills to allow time for preparatory conditioning. Forcing inactive youth to participate in highly competitive sports that are too intense for their current abilities is a losing proposition. Not only will sedentary youth drop out of a sport program such as this, but they will also lose confidence in their abilities to be physically active.

We must also realize that children may not be able to tolerate the same amount of exercise that some of their friends can withstand. This may be particularly important when training adolescents who are experiencing a growth spurt (typically around 12 to 14 years of age). During this time, the relative weakening of the bone, muscle imbalances, and the relative tightening of the muscle tendon units spanning rapidly growing bones are risk factors for overuse injuries. Decreasing the training weight and number of sets performed during periods of rapid growth may be necessary. Thus, we always treat each child as an individual and pay close attention to his or her response to the strength-training program.

important for teachers and coaches to consider the total exercise picture before adding strength training to a child's sport program. Just like other physical activities, strength training contributes to the overall repetitive stress on the young musculoskeletal system, and therefore a teacher or coach must sensibly incorporate strength training into each participant's activity program. Program design considerations for maximizing performance and reducing the risk of overtraining are discussed in chapter 13.

If you incorporate strength training without considering other activities, the overall stress on the growing child may be too great, and the child may experience an overuse injury. We

By enhancing muscular fitness before sport participation, you help aspiring young athletes improve their general athletic skills and reduce their risk of injury. You are also likely to increase their willingness to participate in sport activities.

Being a Teacher

Teachers should be knowledgeable, supportive, and enthusiastic about strength training. They must have a thorough understanding of youth strength-training guidelines and should speak with children at a level the children understand. Teachers should be actively involved in the learning experience and should demonstrate exercises properly. Because children tend to absorb more information with their eyes than with their ears, we keep our verbal instructions short and make a point to demonstrate every exercise to all the children. We often have more experienced boys and girls demonstrate the exercises for the class. This is an important concept because participants who have strength-training experience make good peer tutors, which helps to keep them interested and engaged instead of bored and disruptive.

Teachers should be patient with children and allow them the opportunity to master the performance of an exercise before moving to more advanced training techniques. This is particularly important when working with children who appear physically awkward or clumsy. In this case, provide additional instruction, encouragement, and time to learn a new exercise. In addition, offering these children a choice of exercises might ensure continued participation. For example, if children have difficulty performing a barbell squat exercise, you can suggest a dumbbell squat as an alternative. This would provide an opportunity for the children to continue strength training when they would otherwise be disinterested because of a lack of confidence in their physical abilities. With constructive feedback and adequate time for practice, young people become more confident in their physical abilities and feel more comfortable performing advanced exercises correctly.

> Teachers should be knowledgeable, supportive, and enthusiastic about strength training. They must have a thorough understanding of youth strength-training guidelines and should speak with children at a level the children understand.

We begin our youth strength-training programs with a major focus on education. We do not lecture to children in a classroom, but we do create a learning environment in which participants feel comfortable and capable of succeeding. We spend time discussing safe training procedures, the relevance of strength training, and realistic performance expectations. We remind all participants that it takes time to learn new skills and that long-term progress is made with small gains every training day. Although some young exercisers may want to see how much weight they can lift during the first week of class, we redirect their enthusiasm and interest in strength training toward the development of proper form and technique of a variety of exercises.

We discuss the value of physical activity and introduce the children to proper exercise technique, training guidelines, and safety procedures. Remember show and tell from elementary school? We follow a similar strategy when working with youth. This approach provides a method of teaching strength-training exercises while assessing knowledge, performance, social behaviors, and motivation. After positioning the participants so they all have a clear view of the teacher or coach, we use the following strategy when introducing a new exercise to the class:

1. *Name* the exercise. Use one name and stick with it throughout the lesson.

2. *Explain* the exercise. Use simple terms to describe the exercise and tell the participants how the exercise can benefit them.

3. *Show* the exercise. Demonstrate the exercise several times and from different angles so that all participants can see a full picture of proper execution.

4. *Perform* the exercise. Ask the participants to perform the exercise and offer positive, constructive feedback on proper body position and technique.

5. *Observe* the exercise. Walk around the exercise room and watch the kids strength training. Look for specific skills and ask participants to assess themselves and their peers.

6. *Discuss.* At the end of the session, encourage kids to honestly talk about their perceptions of the day's activities. This

information will help you plan the next session.

Although some participants may want to see how much weight they can lift on the first day of class, we redirect their enthusiasm for strength training by focusing on proper exercise technique. We use checklists that describe in detail proper exercise technique as well as coaching cues. Exercise technique checklists are particularly useful for multijoint lifts such as the squat, bench press, and power clean. Although the amount of weight that participants use for these lifts will vary depending on their body size and strength-training experience, exercise technique checklists can be used for improving exercise form, adjusting training loads, and evaluating individual progress. Figure 3.1 outlines a sample exercise technique checklist for the back squat exercise. This example can be used in creating checklists for other exercises.

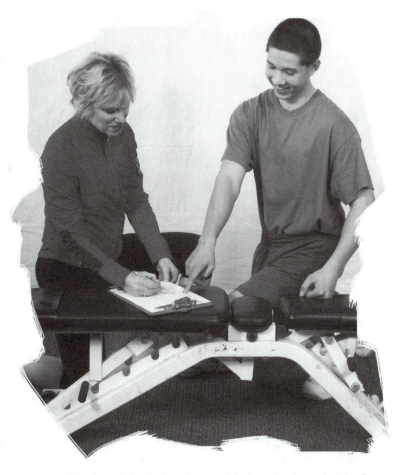

Teach participants how to record their workout on a training log so they can keep track of personal progress.

Developing the Fitness Workout

During the first few training sessions, we develop the concept of a fitness workout that includes dynamic warm-up activities, conditioning exercises, and a cool-down period. While the general format of each lesson is somewhat structured, each class is designed to integrate rather than isolate health- and skill-related fitness components. Combining fitness components is not only more effective and time efficient but is also more enjoyable for children who typically dislike prolonged periods of single-focus training. While there are no shortcuts to developing fundamental fitness skills, this approach to youth fitness has proven to be highly effective.

Along with guidance and encouragement, we teach children how to use training logs so they can record each exercise set and keep track of personal progress. The use of personalized workout logs helps to downplay competition between participants while giving each child's efforts direction and purpose. Workout logs also provide valuable insights into the effectiveness of the strength-training program as well as a child's motivation to exercise. In many cases, a detailed workout log can help the teacher or coach decide when the weight should be increased or when the program should be advanced. Children in our strength-training programs record the weight used, number of sets and repetitions completed, and whether the exercise performance seemed easy or hard. See the sample workout log in appendix A.

Although we are confident that the boys and girls in our programs have learned new physical skills, we are aware of the fact that most participants just want to have fun, build friendships, and feel good about their accomplishments. Children are active like adults, but they are active in different ways and for different reasons. To get a healthy perspective, teachers and coaches sometimes need to remember what they were like as children.

Using Equipment Safely

You need to carefully evaluate the equipment used in your youth strength-training program. Although children can use all types of equipment, they should always follow

EXERCISE: BACK SQUAT

Starting Position

Check

1. Feet are slightly wider than shoulder width and pointing forward or slightly out.   _____

2. Barbell is placed on shoulders and upper back, not on neck.   _____

3. Hands are placed slightly wider than shoulder width.   _____

4. Back is straight; head is in neutral position.   _____

Coaching cue: A spotter should stand directly behind lifter.

Lowering Phase

5. Bar is lowered in a controlled manner.   _____

6. Feet stay flat with heels in contact with floor.   _____

7. Knees follow a slightly outward pattern of the feet; do not let knees cave in.   _____

8. Back stays straight without excessive forward lean.   _____

9. Bar is lowered until thighs are parallel to floor.   _____

Coaching cue: Focus on keeping head up and chest out.

Upward Phase

10. Feet stay flat as bar is raised in a controlled manner.   _____

11. Back stays straight without excessive forward lean.   _____

Coaching cue: Avoid bouncing out of the bottom position.

Finishing Position

12. Knee and hip extension are complete.   _____

13. Barbell is properly returned to rack.   _____

Figure 3.1   An exercise technique checklist for the back squat exercise.

From A. Faigenbaum and W. Westcott, 2009, *Youth Strength Training: Programs for Health, Fitness, and Sport* (Champaign, IL: Human Kinetics).

safety precautions. If we use weight machines, we make sure that each child properly fits onto each machine. Because of variations in body size and shape, it is often necessary to make a few adjustments by adding a pad or changing the position of the resistance lever. As each child grows, you need to make equipment modifications accordingly. It is also important to place the weight machines far enough apart to allow easy access and maneuverability. If children strength train at home, parents need to find safe places to store the weights so younger brothers and sisters don't injure themselves on them.

Parents, teachers, and coaches should take time before every class to ensure that the exercise room is safe and free of clutter. Barbells and dumbbells should be placed on the appropriate racks, and the location of the weight machines should allow for easy access. Overcrowded and poorly designed exercise rooms with too many pieces of equipment increase the likelihood that a child may bump into the equipment or walk into the end of a barbell. Properly designed exercise areas are not only more efficient places to train but are also safer. In addition to developing age-appropriate workouts for young weight trainers,

> Parents, teachers, and coaches should take time before every class to ensure that the exercise room is safe and free of clutter. Barbells and dumbbells should be placed on the appropriate racks, and the location of the weight machines should allow for easy access.

we always design our youth strength-training areas for safe exercise experiences.

We are aware of the exploratory nature of children and therefore remove or disassemble any potential hazards or broken equipment from the exercise room before classes begin. If children use dumbbells or barbells, we always start with a light weight so that they have an opportunity to develop the balance and coordination necessary for performing the exercise correctly. Always teach proper spotting procedures to youth who want to perform free-weight exercises, such as the squat and the bench press. When a child uses dumbbells and barbells, a spotter can help return

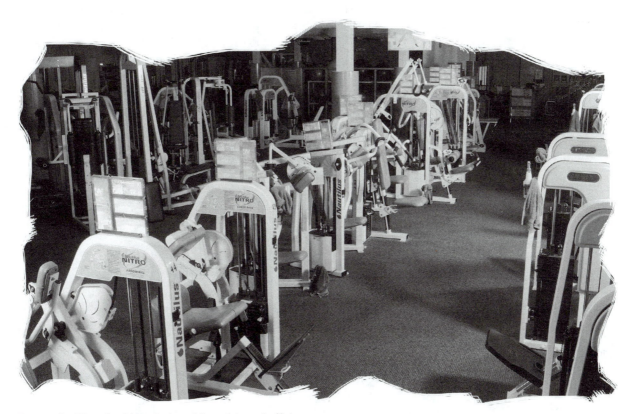

Training facilities should be designed for safety and efficiency.

the weight to the starting position if the child cannot complete the last repetition. If children under the age of 12 perform free-weight exercises such as bench presses that require a spotter, we suggest that a qualified teenager or adult provide the necessary assistance.

Keeping It Progressive

The strength-training program designed for each child should be commensurate with his or her individual abilities. We recognize that children get stronger at different rates and therefore we encourage them to progress at their own pace so they can experience success without injury. Progression to a higher level should be individualized because a variety of factors, including maturation, training age, nutrition, and sleep, can influence the rate at which a child adapts to the training program. Of course, you need to consider the overall ability of the class when working with large groups. In any case, it is important to begin strength training with light loads so that children have an opportunity to develop proper form and technique on each exercise.

Although not every workout needs to be more intense than the previous session, over time the amount of weight lifted should be increased grad-

ually to keep the program fresh and challenging. In most instances a 1- to 5-pound (~0.5 to 2 kg) increase in weight is consistent with a 5 to 10 percent increase in overload. For example, if a child performed 12 repetitions with 50 pounds (~23 kg) on a chest press exercise, he or she should increase the weight to 55 pounds (~25 kg) and decrease repetitions to 8. Although adults may increase their weights by 10 pounds (~5 kg) or more, this is too much for children who typically use less resistance. We also challenge the participants by adding new exercises that require a higher degree of skill yet are attainable with practice. For example, once a participant is able to perform the leg press exercise with proper exercise technique, the performance of the back squat with a lighter load offers a challenging addition to the training program.

Summary

With appropriate guidance and instruction, strength training can become a healthy habit that lasts a lifetime. The key is to understand the uniqueness of children and appreciate the fact that most youth participate in physical activities to learn something new, make friends, and have fun. Take the time to teach children the proper form and technique on each exercise, and be sure to answer any questions they may have. Encourage children to master the performance of basic exercises so they can progress to advanced training techniques. Throughout the program, evaluate each child's responses to the exercise sessions and recognize that children get stronger at different rates. Keeping the fun in fitness will spark an interest in lifelong physical activity.

> Progression to a higher level should be individualized because a variety of factors, including maturation, training age, nutrition, and sleep, can influence the rate at which a child adapts to the training program.

PART II
EXERCISES

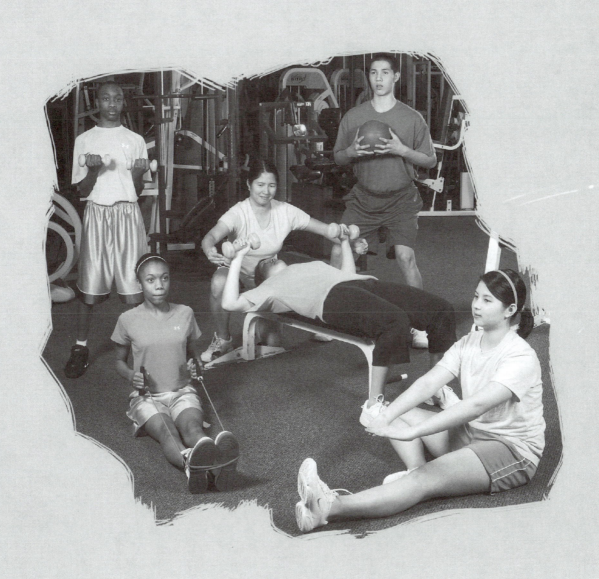

EXERCISES

FREE WEIGHTS

4

The equipment and exercises you will read about in chapters 4, 5, 6, and 7 are only a few of the training options available for your youth strength-training program. We carefully chose several types of training equipment and the best strength-building exercises to provide you with a variety of safe training options. Some exercises require special types of equipment, whereas others don't need any equipment at all. We believe that most modes of strength training can help young people reach their training goals if they perform the exercises correctly. The chapters in part II highlight the advantages and disadvantages of free weights (dumbbells and barbells), weight machines, medicine balls, elastic tubing, and body-weight exercises, including plyometrics. This chapter begins with a discussion on safety, exercise technique, and free-weight training.

Before a child begins lifting weights, the strength-training area must be free of clutter and the room should be well lit and adequately ventilated. The equipment should be in an area that lets children move safely from one station to the next. If free weights are used, benches and weight racks should be nearby so that children do not have to walk too far with weights in their hands. This will decrease traffic flow in the strength-training area. Teachers and coaches also need to designate specific training areas in the weight room for multijoint free-weight lifts. For example, training platforms are ideal for the performance of free-weight exercises such as the power clean and squat because they provide the lifter with enough space to safely perform each exercise. Finally, children should always return barbells and dumbbells to the appropriate racks so they don't slip or trip on them. Following these safety guidelines can reduce the likelihood of injuries occurring in the weight-training area.

When teaching a child a strength-training exercise, always focus on form and technique rather than the amount of weight he or she lifts. Thus, you must completely understand how to perform an exercise before attempting to teach it to a child. Work with children in small groups, and always encourage children to ask questions and comment on the program. When teaching children a new exercise, demonstrate five or six repetitions of the exercise, highlighting the muscles used, the importance of controlled movements throughout a full range of motion, correct body positioning, and proper breathing (exhale during the lifting phase and inhale during the lowering phase). When teaching children a free-weight exercise, always start with a light weight, wooden stick, or PVC pipe. This helps participants focus on form and technique while minimizing muscle soreness.

When a child performs a new exercise, provide constructive feedback regarding the child's exercise performance, and gratefully acknowledge the child's willingness to demonstrate an exercise in front of his or her peers. Realizing that learning most free-weight exercises requires coordination and concentration, limit the number of new exercises you add to a child's routine on any day. From our experience, attempting to add too many exercises to a child's routine at one time slows the learning process and takes some fun out of the exercise program. Teach children something new every session so that they want to lift weights when they come to your class and therefore spend most of the time enjoying the exercises.

When you teach children free-weight exercises, remember to demonstrate proper spotting techniques, which are essential for safe free-weight training. A spotter is a safety person who should be nearby to assist when a child is lifting a weight over the body, when loss of balance might occur, or when a child is learning a new exercise. Spotters should know proper exercise technique and should be able to handle the weight the child is lifting in case he or she needs assistance. Spotters should communicate with the lifters and should know how many repetitions the lifter will complete. Teachers and coaches need to demonstrate and explain proper spotting techniques because the purpose of correct spotting is to prevent injury. If children are too young to spot each other or if they have special needs and are unable to provide the necessary assistance, adults or teenagers with training experience should serve as spotters. When working with a large class of children, it might be necessary to enlist the help of additional adults or separate the class into small groups.

In some cases, teachers and coaches need to be aware of the considerable amount of time it takes to learn an advanced lift and should be knowledgeable of the stepwise progression from basic exercises to more advanced movements. For example, total-body power exercises such as the power clean, snatch, and push press are explosive but highly controlled movements that require far more technical skill than basic strength exercises such as the leg extension and biceps curl. Thus, youth should perform fewer repetitions (about 6 to 8) on a power exercise compared to a strength exercise because every repetition of a power exercise should be performed with vigor. Clearly, youth need time to develop the skill, technique, and confidence to perform total-body power exercises correctly and need to understand safety procedures. For example, all young lifters should learn how to properly return the barbell to the floor if an advanced lift cannot be performed correctly. By practicing how to "miss" a lift with a wooden dowel or PVC rod, youth become automatic in their responses to an undesirable bar position.

Various training modalities have proven safe and effective. Nevertheless, we all need to appreciate that improper exercise technique on any type of equipment can place undue stress on a body part and might result in injury. This is an important consideration when performing free-weight exercises. For example, a child can injure the lower back if he or she does a rocking motion when performing a simple exercise such as the barbell curl. If this happens, it usually means that the child is lifting too much weight or isn't paying attention to the proper exercise technique. Without competent supervision and instruction, children can develop poor exercise habits and injure themselves. You need to be sure that children understand the benefits as well as the risks inherent in this type of training. Constantly emphasize safety, and under no circumstances allow horseplay in the strength-training area. In our programs, all teachers and coaches demonstrate their commitment to safe strength training through their own actions in the strength-training area.

Training With Free Weights

Free-weight training refers to using barbells and dumbbells as well as various types of benches and racks. Barbells and dumbbells come in various shapes and sizes and may be adjustable or

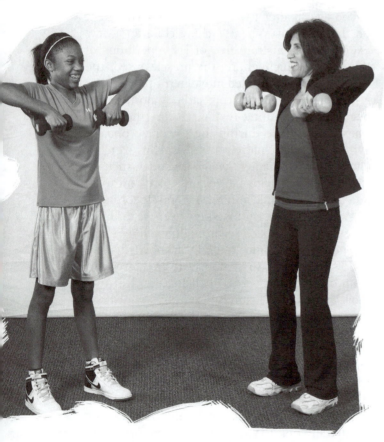

Focus on proper technique rather than the amount of weight lifted.

fixed. Most barbells sold in sporting good stores are about 5 feet long (1.5 m) and weigh about 15 to 25 pounds (~7 to 11 kg). Olympic-style barbells, which have sleeves on each end that allow the bar to revolve during a lift, are about 7 feet long (2 m) and weigh 45 pounds (20 kg). Lighter-weight Olympic-style aluminum barbells that weigh 15 pounds (~7 kg) as well as 5-pound (2 kg) plastic training plates are also available and can be very useful for teaching youth free-weight exercises.

The adjustable barbells and dumbbells enable you to change the weight as needed by adding or removing weight plates, which you can secure to the bar by collars or locks. On the other hand, fixed barbells and dumbbells come in a predetermined weight that you cannot change. Because you don't have to change the weight for each exercise, fixed free weights can decrease the time of your workout. However, you will need to purchase several of them for all the exercises in a workout. Depending on the age and ability of the children, these could include pairs of 2-, 3-, 5-, 8-, and 10-pound dumbbells (~1, 1.5, 2, 3.5, and 5 kg). An economical approach is to purchase two adjustable dumbbells and several weight plates that are appropriate for each child's training level. Whatever type of equipment you use, keep in mind that it is important to increase the weight gradually as a child gets stronger. Generally, we use 1-, 3-, or 5-pound increases depending on the exercise. For example, a 1-pound increase may be appropriate for a single-joint exercise such as the biceps curl, whereas a 5-pound increase may be reasonable for a multijoint exercise such as the back squat.

Although most free-weight exercises described in this chapter require only dumbbells or barbells, some free-weight exercises are performed on a weight bench in a sitting or lying position. Weight benches are typically of two types: flat and incline. The adjustable-incline weight bench is the most versatile because you can change it to various angles and seat positions. For general conditioning, any type of flat weight bench can work. You will also need equipment such as a squat rack if you decide to perform exercises such as the back squat or front squat. Lifting platforms may also be needed for advanced free-weight exercises. While some high schools have official weightlifting platforms, others construct platforms from wood and install thick rubber mats where weights will be placed on the floor.

Free weights are inexpensive and do not take up much room. Since barbells and dumbbells allow unrestrained movement patterns, a person can perform all free-weight exercises throughout their full ranges of motion. In addition, if one side of a child's body is weaker than the other, free weights allow for the restoration of muscle balance with appropriate training. Another advantage of using free weights over other types of equipment is that children of all sizes can use them and can perform hundreds of exercises, including total-body movements. This helps to improve muscle coordination because a child must learn to balance the weight in all directions (up, down, left, and right). Well-coached youth who gain confidence and skill in performing total-body movements will be better prepared for more advanced strength and conditioning programs that include traditional weightlifting movements, such as the power clean and snatch.

> Free weights are inexpensive and do not take up much room. Since barbells and dumbbells allow unrestrained movement patterns, a person can perform all free-weight exercises throughout their full ranges of motion.

In general, you can consider free-weight training more technical than other modes of training, and therefore you must emphasize proper instruction and close supervision to be sure that the children perform the exercises correctly. Because the movements are not fixed (as on weight machines), children may need more time to learn the proper exercise technique. You also need to teach children how to hold dumbbells and weight plates correctly so that they don't slip and fall out of their hands. During the first exercise session, you should teach children how to hold free weights correctly with the thumb hooked around the dumbbell or barbell.

It is also important to teach children about spotting, which is the practice of assisting a lifter if an exercise cannot be completed. Spotters can also provide feedback regarding safety and

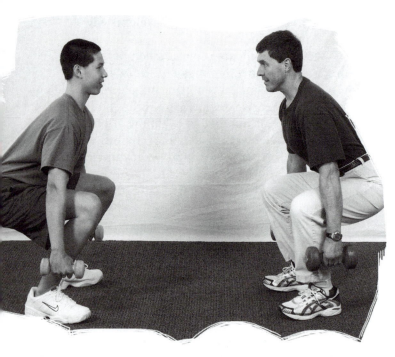

Always demonstrate correct body positioning when teaching a free-weight exercise.

correct exercise technique. For example, spotters should ensure that the barbell is evenly loaded and the weights are secured with collars. Obviously, spotters must be aware of proper exercise technique and must be strong enough to assist the lifters in case of a failed repetition. If children with limited strength-training experience are not capable of spotting each other, an adult or a more experienced lifter should serve as the spotter. Although a spotter is not needed for all free-weight exercises, barbell exercises such as the bench press and squat are commonly spotted by people with strength-training experience. Exercises such as the dumbbell curl or deadlift do not require a spotter because the lifter can safely lower the weight to the floor if he or she cannot complete a repetition with proper exercise technique.

Children also need to focus on the development of abdominal and lower-back strength. This concern is important not only for sedentary children who typically have weak supporting muscles in their torsos, but also for youth who want to perform free-weight exercises such as the squat. Our program begins with exercises for the abdominal muscles and lower back as well as exercises for the legs, chest, back, and arms. Over time we progress to advanced lifting techniques

based on a child's exercise performance and willingness to try more challenging lifts.

Free-Weight Exercises

The free-weight exercises are organized into three major sections: upper body, lower body, and total body. Included are lists of the specific names of the primary muscle groups strengthened by each upper- and lower-body exercise. Understanding the muscles that you are training will help you design a balanced strength-training program. For example, overexercising the quadriceps (muscles on the front of the thigh) and underexercising the hamstrings (muscles on the back of the thigh) may increase a child's risk of injury. Children should strength train all the major muscle groups to get the most benefit from their workouts. Be sure to follow these safety guidelines when training children and adolescents with free weights:

- Enlist knowledgeable adults who provide careful instruction and close supervision.
- Load dumbbells and barbells evenly and secure the weight plates with safety collars.
- Check the stability of training platforms, benches and racks before you use them.
- Use a spotter who can assist in case of a failed repetition when doing squats, bench presses, and incline presses.
- Begin each exercise with a relatively light weight and focus on learning the correct form of each exercise.
- Terminate any exercise that is not being performed with proper technique.
- Remove weights from the floor to prevent slipping or tripping.
- Secure the training room when not in use to prevent unauthorized use of exercise equipment.

Understanding the muscles that you are training will help you design a balanced strength-training program.

DUMBBELL CHEST PRESS

Muscles

Pectoralis major, anterior deltoid, triceps

Procedure

1. Grasp a dumbbell in each hand. Lie on your back on a bench with your feet flat on the floor. If your feet don't reach the floor, use a stable board to accommodate size. Hold the dumbbells at arm's length over the chest area with palms facing away from your body.

2. Slowly bend your elbows and lower the dumbbells to the outside of the chest area.

3. Press the dumbbells upward until you fully extend both arms.

Technique Tips

- Keep your head, shoulders, and buttocks in contact with the bench during this exercise. Do not twist or arch your body.

- Keep the dumbbells above your chest and not above your face.

- It is important that a spotter be nearby to provide assistance if needed. A spotter can place his or her hands on the child's wrists to teach proper dumbbell exercise technique or complete a repetition.

- You can also perform this exercise with a barbell, provided that skilled instruction and supervision are available. If you perform this exercise with a barbell, an adult spotter must be nearby to provide assistance if necessary.

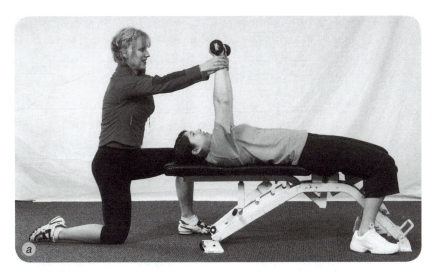

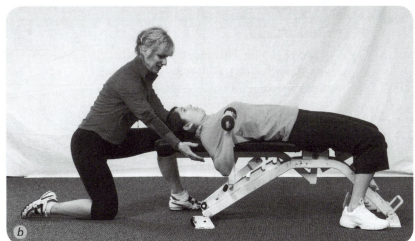

BARBELL BENCH PRESS

Muscles

Pectoralis major, anterior deltoid, triceps

Procedure

1. Lie on your back with your feet flat on the floor. If your feet don't reach the floor, use a stable board to accommodate size. Grasp the barbell with a wider than shoulder-width grip, wrapping thumbs around the bar. Hold the barbell at arm's length above your upper-chest area.

2. Slowly lower the barbell to the middle of your chest. In the bottom position the forearms should be perpendicular to the floor. Pause briefly, then press the barbell to the starting position. During the movement, the upper arms should be about 45 to 60 degrees from the torso and the hips should remain on the bench.

Technique Tips

- A spotter should be behind the lifter's head and should assist the lifter with getting the barbell into the starting position and returning the barbell to the rack when finished. Impress on young weight trainers the importance of a spotter during the exercise because the bar is pressed over the lifter's face, neck, and chest.

- Learn this exercise with an unloaded barbell or light weight.

- Do not bounce the barbell off the chest, and do not lift your buttocks off the bench during this exercise.

- To avoid hitting the upright supports, position your shoulders at least 3 inches (~8 cm) from the supports before you start.

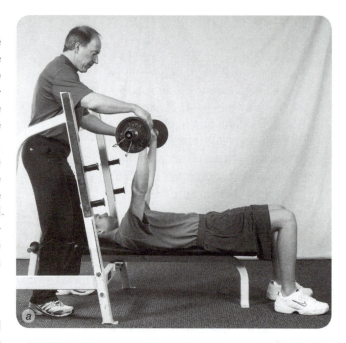

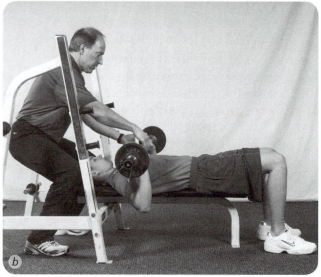

DUMBBELL INCLINE PRESS

Muscles

Pectoralis major, anterior deltoid, triceps

Procedure

1. Grasp a dumbbell in each hand. Lie on your back on an incline bench (30- to 45-degree angle) with your feet flat on the floor. If your feet don't reach the floor, use a stable board to accommodate size. Hold the dumbbells at arm's length over the shoulder and upper-chest area with palms facing away from your body.

2. Slowly bend your elbows and lower the dumbbells to the outside of the upper-chest area.

3. Press the dumbbells upward until you fully extend both arms.

Technique Tips

- Keep your head, shoulders, and buttocks in contact with the bench during this exercise. Do not twist or arch your body.

- Keep the dumbbells above the shoulder and chest area and not above your face.

- It is important that a spotter be nearby to provide assistance if needed. A spotter can place his or her hands on the child's wrists to teach proper dumbbell exercise technique or complete a repetition.

- You can also perform this exercise with a barbell, provided that skilled instruction and supervision are available. If you perform this exercise with a barbell, an adult spotter must be nearby to provide assistance if necessary.

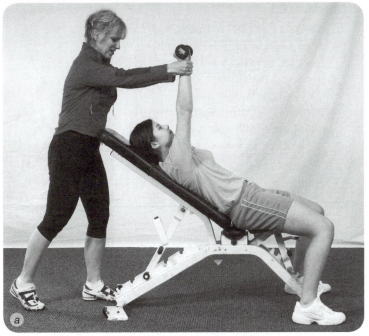

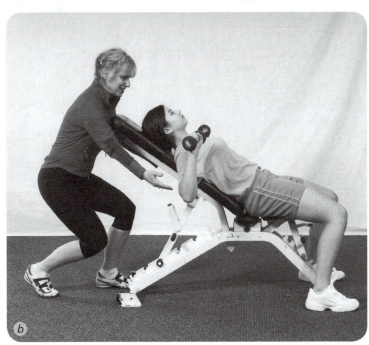

DUMBBELL CHEST FLY

Muscles

Pectoralis major, anterior deltoid

Procedure

1. Grasp a dumbbell in each hand. Lie on your back on a bench with your feet flat on the floor. If your feet don't reach the floor, use a stable lift to accommodate size. Hold the dumbbells at arm's length over the chest area with your palms facing each other and arms slightly bent.

2. Slowly lower the dumbbells until your upper arms are parallel to the floor. You should feel a gentle stretch across your chest.

3. Lift the dumbbells to starting position, keeping your elbows slightly bent.

Technique Tips

- Keep head, shoulders, and buttocks in contact with the bench during this exercise. Do not twist or arch your body.

- Keep the dumbbells above your chest and not above your face.

- Do not lower dumbbells below parallel to the floor because this will place increased stress on the shoulder joint.

- It is important that a spotter be nearby to provide assistance if needed. A spotter can place his or her hands on the child's wrists to teach proper exercise technique or complete a repetition.

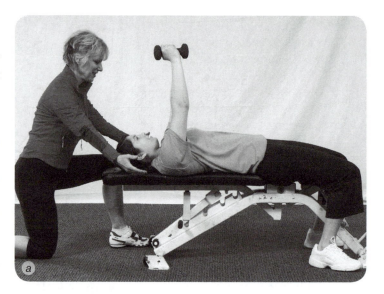

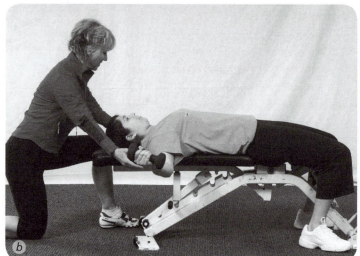

DUMBBELL ONE-ARM ROW

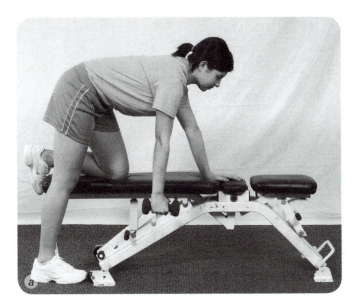
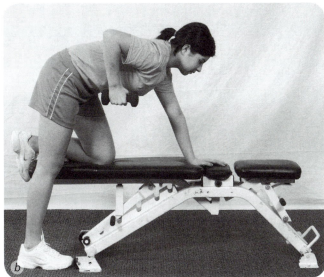

Muscles

Latissimus dorsi, biceps

Procedure

1. Grasp a dumbbell in the right hand with the palm facing the side of the body, and place the left hand and left knee on the bench. Bend over at the waist so the upper body and lower back are parallel to the floor (i.e., flat). Support the body on the bench, and keep the back flat from the shoulders to the hips. Lower the dumbbell toward the floor so you fully extend the right arm.

2. Slowly pull the dumbbell upward until it reaches the side of the chest area. Then lower the dumbbell back to the straight-arm position. Perform the assigned number of repetitions; then switch the supporting posture and perform the exercise on your left side.

Technique Tips

- The legs and nonexercising arm should remain stationary during the exercise. The lower back should not rotate during this exercise.
- For a variation, you can perform this exercise with the elbow pointing away from the body (palm toward feet) during the lifting motion.

DUMBBELL PULLOVER

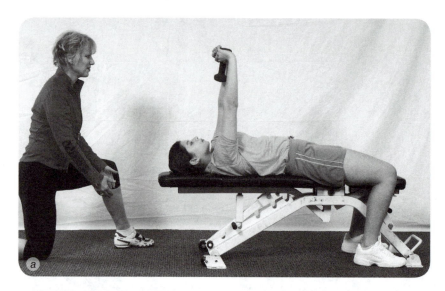

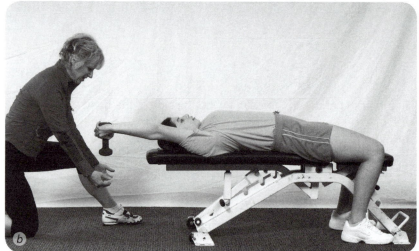

Muscle

Latissimus dorsi

Procedure

1. Grasp one dumbbell with both hands, and lie on a flat bench with your arms extended over your chest area. Secure your grip by cupping both hands around one end of the dumbbell.

2. Leading with the elbows, slowly lower the dumbbell behind your head toward the floor as far as comfortable. Maintain a slight bend in your elbows. Then slowly return to starting position.

Technique Tips

- A spotter should kneel directly behind the lifter's head during this exercise and provide assistance if necessary.

- Because the dumbbell is over the head of the lifter, begin with a light weight and gradually increase the load. We recommend a solid dumbbell (rather than a dumbbell with plates and collars) for this exercise.

DUMBBELL UPRIGHT ROW

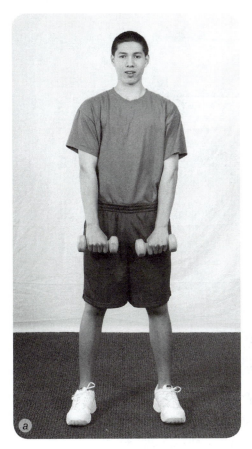 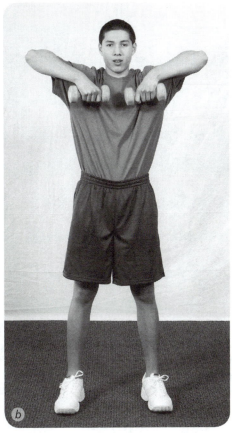

Muscles

Deltoids, upper trapezius, biceps

Procedure

1. Begin by grasping a dumbbell in each hand, and stand erect with feet about hip-width apart. Hold the dumbbells so they hang straight down in front of your body with your palms facing your body. The dumbbells should be closer than shoulder-width apart.

2. Slowly pull both dumbbells upward to the height of the upper chest; then lower them to the starting position.

Technique Tips

- Stand erect and keep the dumbbells close to your body during this exercise.

- At the top of the movement, the elbows should be higher than the shoulders.

- You can also perform this exercise with a barbell, provided that skilled instruction and supervision are available.

DUMBBELL OVERHEAD PRESS

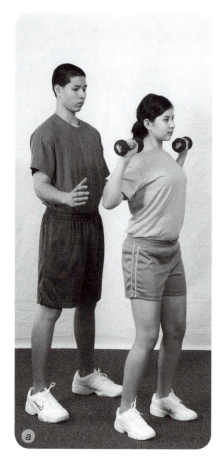 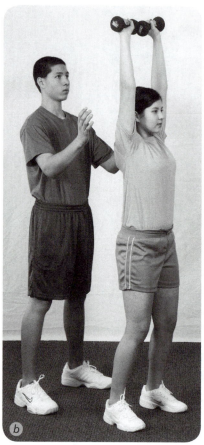

Muscles

Deltoids, upper trapezius, triceps

Procedure

1. Begin by grasping a dumbbell in each hand, and stand erect with feet about hip-width apart. Hold the dumbbells at shoulder height with your palms facing away from your body.

2. Slowly push both dumbbells upward until you fully extend both arms over the shoulders; then lower the dumbbells to the starting position.

Technique Tips

- This exercise requires balance and coordination. Begin with a light weight to learn proper form.

- Stand erect and keep your lower back straight by contracting your abdominal and lower-back muscles.

- You can also perform this exercise while sitting on an adjustable-incline bench or chair, which can provide back support and stability.

- You can also perform this exercise with a barbell, provided that skilled instruction and supervision are available.

- It is important that a spotter be nearby to provide assistance if needed. A spotter can place his or her hands on the child's wrists to teach proper exercise technique or complete a repetition.

DUMBBELL LATERAL RAISE

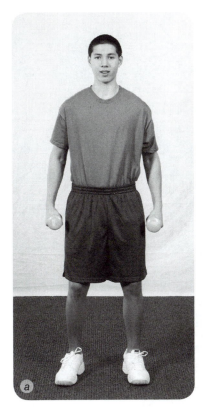 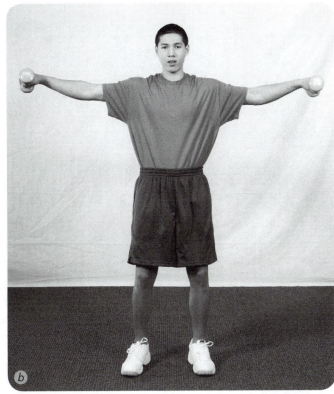

Muscle
Deltoids

Procedure

1. Begin by grasping a dumbbell in each hand, and stand erect with your arms extended at your sides and palms facing your outer thighs. Your elbows should be slightly bent, and your feet should be about hip-width apart.

2. Slowly lift both dumbbells upward and sideward until your arms are level with your shoulders (arms parallel to floor). Keep your elbows slightly bent, and return to starting position.

Technique Tips

- Stand erect and keep your lower back straight by contracting your abdominal and lower-back muscles.
- Avoid leaning backward.
- Don't raise your arms higher than parallel to the floor.

DUMBBELL SHRUG

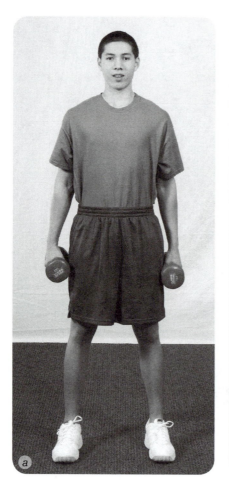
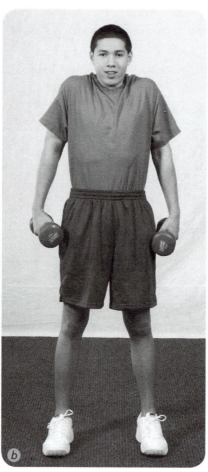

Muscle
Upper trapezius

Procedure
1. Begin by grasping a dumbbell in each hand, and stand erect with your arms extended at your sides, palms facing your outer thighs, and head straight. Your arms should be fully extended, and your feet should be about hip-width apart.
2. Slowly elevate (shrug) both shoulders toward the ears as high as possible; then lower both dumbbells to the starting position.

Technique Tips
- Stand erect and keep your lower back straight by contracting your abdominal and lower-back muscles.
- Don't bend your elbows while lifting the weights.

DUMBBELL EXTERNAL ROTATION

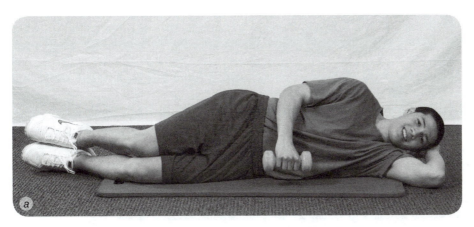

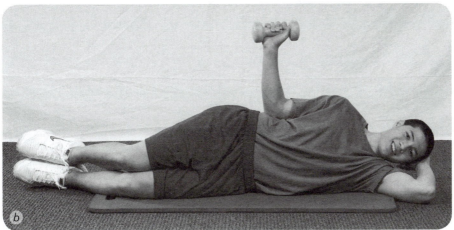

Muscle

Rotator cuff musculature

Procedure

1. Lie on your side in a comfortable position. Hold a light dumbbell with the top hand, and maintain the elbow at a 90-degree angle. Hold the upper arm against the side of your body. Use your other arm to support your head.

2. Rotate your forearm out and up without letting your elbow move away from your body. Then slowly return to the starting position.

Technique Tips

- This is a lightweight exercise with a limited range of motion. Start with a 2- or 3-pound dumbbell (1 to 1.5 kg), and increase in 1-pound (0.5 kg) increments.

- Keep your arm pressed against your body during this exercise.

- You can also perform this exercise in the standing position by using elastic tubing attached to a sturdy object or a cable attached to appropriate resistance.

DUMBBELL SHOULDER INTERNAL ROTATION

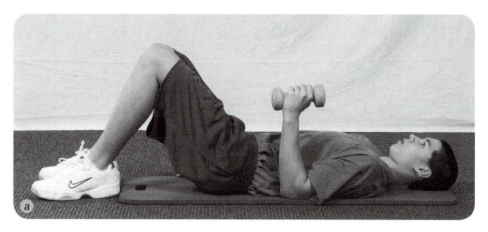

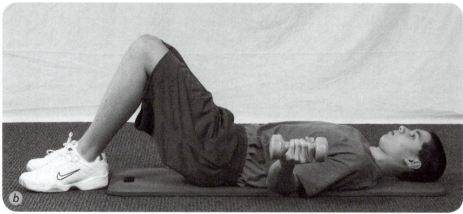

Muscle

Rotator cuff musculature

Procedure

1. Lie on your back in a comfortable position. Hold a light dumbbell with one hand, and maintain the elbow at a 90-degree angle. Hold your upper arm on the floor against the side of your body and your forearm perpendicular to the floor.

2. Slowly lower the dumbbell toward the floor by rotating your shoulder. Then return to the starting position.

Technique Tips

- This is a lightweight exercise with a limited range of motion. Start with a 2- or 3-pound dumbbell (1 or 1.5 kg), and increase in 1-pound (0.5 kg) increments.

- Keep the elbow pressed against your body during this exercise.

- You can also perform this exercise in the standing position by using elastic tubing attached to a sturdy object or a cable attached to appropriate resistance.

DUMBBELL BICEPS CURL

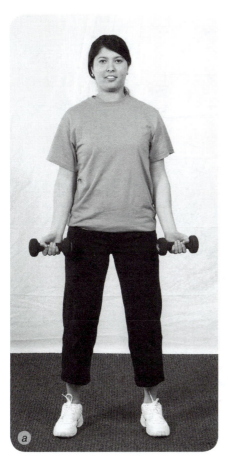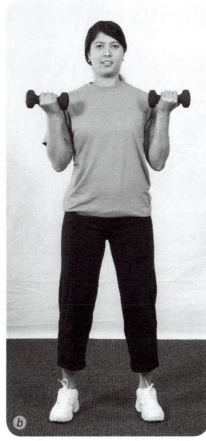

Muscle
Biceps

Procedure
1. Begin by grasping a dumbbell in each hand, and stand erect with your arms extended at your sides and palms facing forward. Fully extend your arms, and place your feet about hip-width apart.
2. Slowly curl one dumbbell upward toward your shoulders until your palm faces the chest. Then lower the dumbbell to the starting position and repeat with the other arm.

Technique Tips
- Stand erect with knees slightly bent and keep your lower back straight by contracting your abdominal and lower-back muscles.
- If necessary, stand with your back against the wall to prevent upper-body movement.
- You can also perform this exercise while sitting on an adjustable-incline bench, which can provide back support and stability.
- As an alternative, perform this exercise with a barbell or lift each dumbbell alternately rather than in unison.

DUMBBELL INCLINE BICEPS CURL

This exercise is the same as the dumbbell biceps curl, except you perform it on an incline bench, typically angled between 45 and 60 degrees.

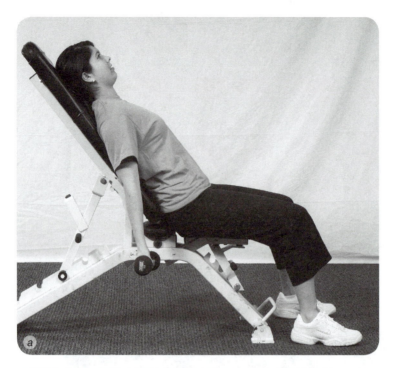

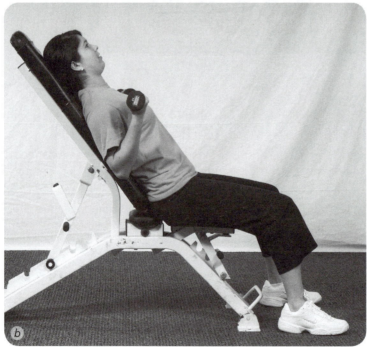

DUMBBELL HAMMER CURL

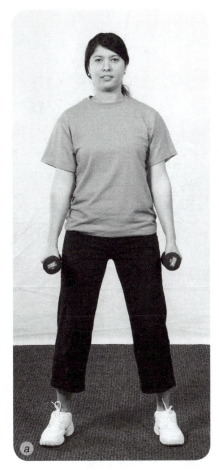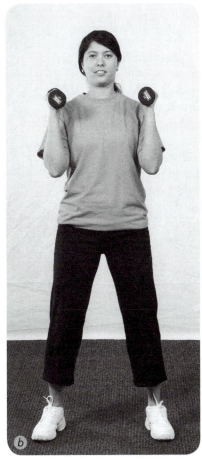

Muscles

Biceps, brachioradialis

Procedure

1. Begin by grasping a dumbbell in each hand, and stand erect with your arms extended at your sides and palms facing inward. Fully extend your arms with the dumbbells alongside the thighs, and place your feet about hip-width apart with knees slightly bent.

2. Slowly curl both dumbbells upward toward your shoulder with your palm facing your torso. Then lower the dumbbells to the starting position and repeat.

Technique Tips

- Stand erect and keep your lower back straight by contracting your abdominal and lower-back muscles.

- If necessary, stand with your back against the wall to prevent upper-body movement.

- You can also perform this exercise while sitting on an adjustable-incline bench, which can provide back support and stability.

- As an alternative, perform this exercise with a barbell or lift each dumbbell alternately rather than in unison.

DUMBBELL TRICEPS KICKBACK

Muscle
Triceps

Procedure

1. Grasp a dumbbell in the right hand with the palm facing the side of the body, and place the left hand and left knee on the bench. Bend over at the waist so the upper body and lower back are parallel to the floor (i.e., flat). Bend the right elbow to 90 degrees so the upper arm is against the side and the right forearm is perpendicular to the floor. Support the body on the bench, and keep the back flat from the shoulders to the hips.

2. Slowly straighten the right arm until it is fully extended; then return to the starting position. Perform the assigned number of repetitions; then switch your supporting posture and perform the exercise with your left arm.

Technique Tip
Only the elbow and forearm should move during this exercise. The legs and nonexercising arm should remain stationary and the lower back should not rotate.

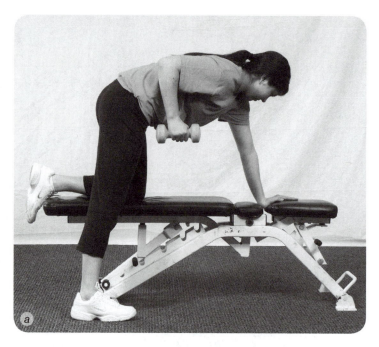

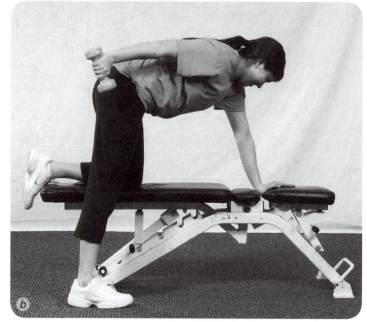

DUMBBELL WRIST CURL

Muscle

Wrist flexor

Procedure

1. Begin by kneeling on the floor with the forearms resting on a bench. Grasp a dumbbell in each hand in a palms-up position so the wrists hang just over the bench.

2. Slowly flex the fingers and the wrists as high as possible while keeping the forearms flat on the bench; then return to starting position.

Technique Tips

- The entire forearm should remain in contact with the bench during this exercise. Only the fingers and wrists should move.

- You can also perform this exercise with one dumbbell at a time or with a barbell.

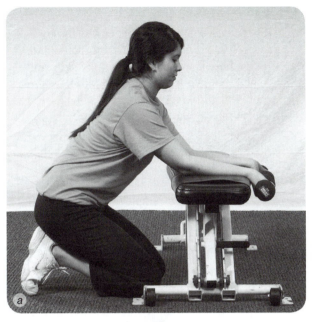

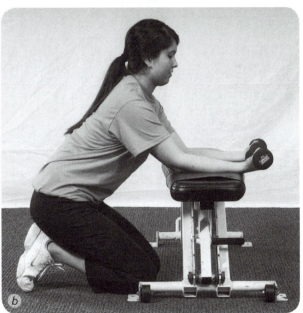

DUMBBELL WRIST EXTENSION

Muscle
Wrist extensor

Procedure
1. Begin by kneeling on the floor with the forearms resting on a bench. Grasp a dumbbell in each hand in a palms-down position, and place the palm side of the forearms on the bench so the wrists hang just over the bench.
2. Slowly lift the fingers and the wrists as high as possible while keeping the forearms flat on the bench; then return to starting position.

Technique Tips
• The entire forearm should remain in contact with the bench during this exercise. Only the fingers and wrists should move.

• Because this muscle group is relatively weak, begin with a light weight.

• You can also perform this exercise with one dumbbell at a time or with a barbell.

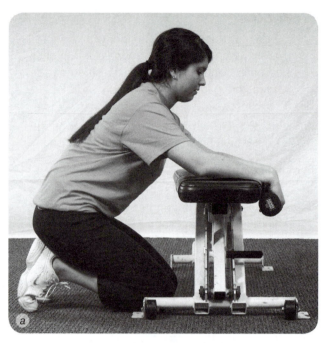

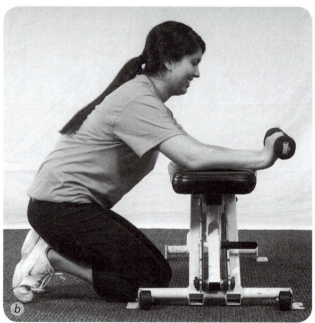

WRIST ROLLER

Muscles

Wrist flexors and extensors

Procedure

1. Grasp the handle of the wrist roller with your palms facing downward. Stand erect with your elbows bent slightly.
2. Roll up the string on the bar until the weight reaches the uppermost point. Then slowly unroll the string.

Technique Tips

- Start with a light weight, and gradually increase the resistance as strength improves.
- Vary the exercise by starting with the string between you and the roller and with the string on the opposite side of the roller.
- As you rotate the roller clockwise, you strengthen the wrist flexors. As you rotate the roller counterclockwise, you strengthen the wrist extensors.

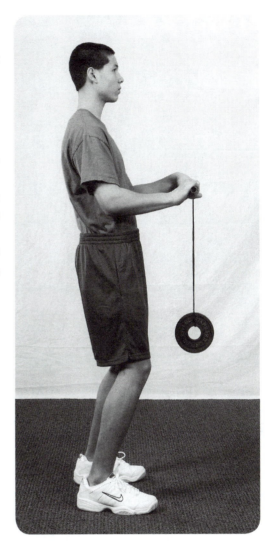

DUMBBELL SQUAT

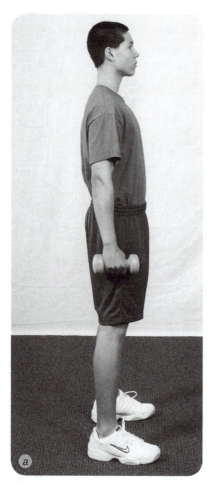
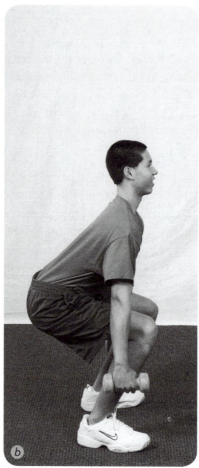

Muscles

Quadriceps, gluteals, hamstrings, erector spinae

Procedure

1. Begin by grasping a dumbbell in each hand, and stand erect with feet about shoulder-width apart and toes pointing slightly outward. Hold the dumbbells so they hang straight down at the sides of your body with palms facing thighs.

2. Slowly move hips backward and then immediately bend at the knees until your thighs are parallel to the floor. Keep your back flat, head up, and heels in contact with the floor and knees over the toes.

3. Return to starting position by slowly straightening your knees and hips.

Technique Tips

- Your knees should follow a slightly outward pattern of the feet. Do not let the knees cave in.
- Avoid bouncing out of the bottom position.
- Concentrate on keeping your head up and chest out. Avoid excessive forward lean.
- You can perform partial repetitions if you cannot reach the thigh-parallel-to-the-floor position with proper form.

BARBELL BACK SQUAT

Muscles
Quadriceps, gluteals, hamstrings, erector spinae

Procedure

1. Grasp the barbell with an overhand grip while it is on the rack.

2. Your hands should be wider than shoulder-width apart, and the barbell should rest on your shoulders and upper trapezius muscle, not on your neck.

3. Lift the bar off the rack. Keep your back straight, eyes focused forward, and feet slightly wider than shoulder-width apart with toes pointing slightly outward.

4. Slowly move hips backward and then immediately bend at the knees until your thighs are parallel to the floor. Keep your heels in contact with the floor and your knees over the toes.

5. Return to the starting position by straightening your hips and knees. Do not allow the hips to rise faster than the bar during the upward movement phase.

6. When you have completed the desired number of repetitions, walk the barbell back to the rack.

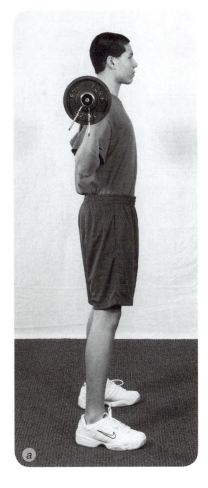
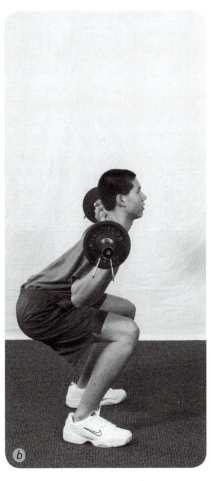

Technique Tips

- Your back should remain upright during this exercise. Excessive forward lean places undue stress on your lower back and may result in an injury.

- A spotter should stand directly behind you during this exercise.

- You can perform partial repetitions if you cannot reach the thigh-parallel-to-the-floor position with proper form.

BARBELL FRONT SQUAT

Muscles

Quadriceps, gluteals, hamstrings, erector spinae

Procedure

1. Grasp the barbell with a grip slightly wider than shoulder width while it is on the rack. Let the shoulders come forward to create a shelf for the bar in front of the body.

2. Lift the bar off the rack. Keep your back straight, eyes focused forward, and feet slightly wider than shoulder-width apart with toes pointing slightly outward.

3. Slowly move hips backward and then immediately bend at the knees until your thighs are parallel to the floor. Keep your heels in contact with the floor and your knees over the toes.

4. Return to the starting position by straightening your hips and knees. Do not allow the hips to rise faster than the bar during the upward movement phase.

5. When you have completed the desired number of repetitions, walk the barbell back to the rack.

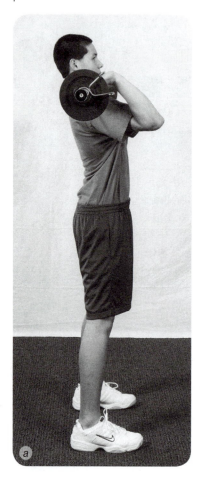
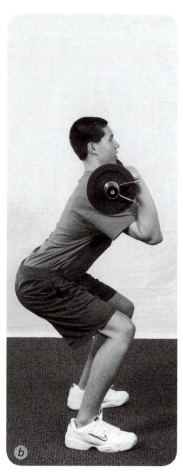

Technique Tips

- Your back should remain upright during this exercise. Excessive forward lean places undue stress on your lower back and may result in an injury.

- A spotter should stand directly behind the lifter during this exercise.

- You can perform partial repetitions if you cannot reach the thigh-parallel-to-the-floor position with proper form.

BARBELL DEADLIFT

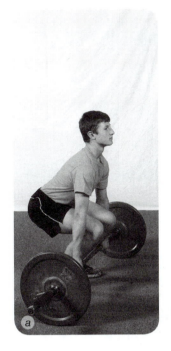 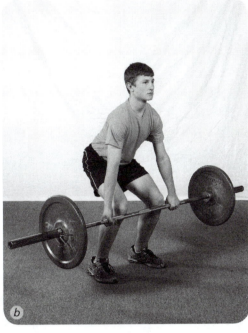 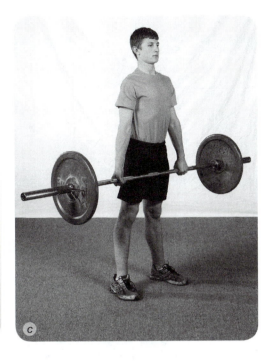

Muscles

Quadriceps, gluteals, hamstrings, erector spinae

Procedure

1. Stand behind barbell with feet shoulder-width apart. Bend hips and knees and grasp the barbell with one underhand and one overhand grip with arms extended, hands slightly wider than shoulder width, and hips lower than shoulders. Torso should be at 45 degrees.

2. Using the legs, lift the barbell off the floor to the knees while maintaining torso at 45 degrees. Move to an upright position when bar reaches top of knees.

3. Return to the starting position by bending your hips and knees.

Technique Tips

- During the initial phase of the lift, keep the hips low and chest up.
- Maintain a flat back position throughout this exercise. Do not bend the torso forward.
- Learn proper technique with a wooden dowel or light barbell.
- This exercise can be performed with dumbbells as an alternative.

DUMBBELL LUNGE

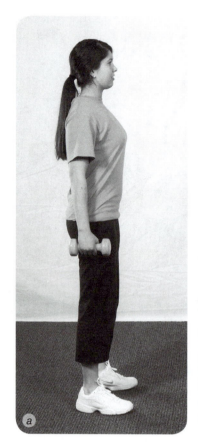 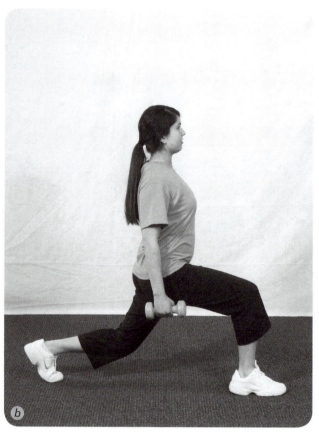

Muscles

Quadriceps, hamstrings, gluteals

Procedure

1. Begin by grasping a dumbbell in each hand. Stand erect with feet about hip-width apart, and hold the dumbbells so that they hang straight down at the sides of your body. Look straight forward.

2. Take a long step forward with your right leg; bend the knee of the right leg and lower your body. The thigh of the right leg should be parallel to the floor, and the right knee should be over the ankle of the right foot. Bend the left knee slightly.

3. Return to the starting position by pushing off the floor with the right leg. Take one or two steps backward to the starting position. Repeat with the opposite leg.

4. Keep your head up, back upright, and shoulders over hips.

Technique Tips

- This exercise requires balance and coordination. Begin with just your body weight to learn proper form.

- Keep your head up, back upright, and shoulders over hips.

- Avoid using upper-torso momentum to return to the starting position. Concentrate on keeping your back upright throughout the exercise.

DUMBBELL SIDE LUNGE

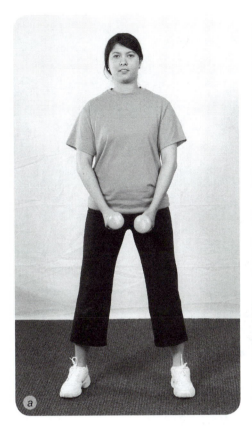

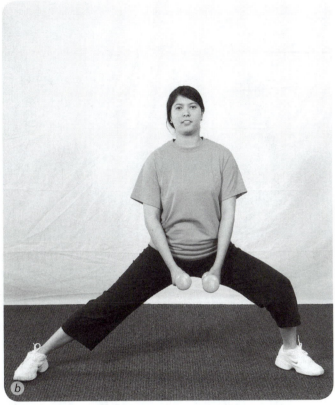

Muscles

Quadriceps, hamstrings, gluteals, hip abductors and adductors

Procedure

1. Begin by grasping a dumbbell in each hand. Stand erect with your feet about shoulder-width apart, and hold the dumbbells in front of your body. Look straight forward.
2. Step to the side with one leg while holding the dumbbells in front of your body. The stepping leg should be at a 45-degree angle to the body.
3. Point your toes slightly to the side as you step out.
4. Bend your knee until your thigh is parallel to the floor.
5. Push yourself to the starting position.
6. Repeat with the opposite leg.

Technique Tips

- Keep your head up and facing forward during this exercise.
- This exercise requires balance and coordination. To learn the proper form, begin with just your body weight.

DUMBBELL STEP-UP

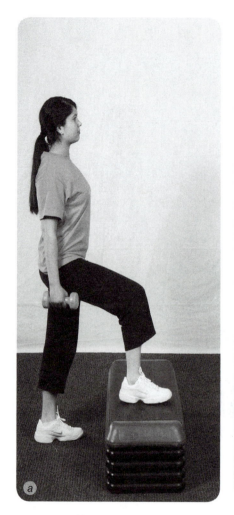
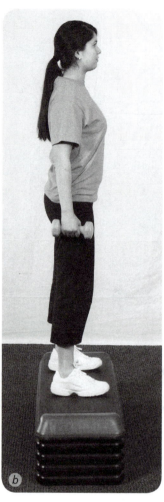

Muscles

Quadriceps, gluteals, hamstrings

Procedure

1. Begin by grasping a dumbbell in each hand, and stand erect with feet about hip-width apart. Hold the dumbbells so that they hang straight down at your sides. Look straight forward.

2. Step with your right leg onto a bench that is about knee height. Lift your body with your right leg. Bring your left knee up.

3. Slowly lower your body by stepping back down to the starting position. Repeat with the opposite leg.

Technique Tips

- This exercise requires balance and coordination. To learn proper form, begin with just your body weight.

- Concentrate on keeping the torso upright during this exercise.

- Before starting, check to be sure the bench is stable and secure.

DUMBBELL HEEL RAISE

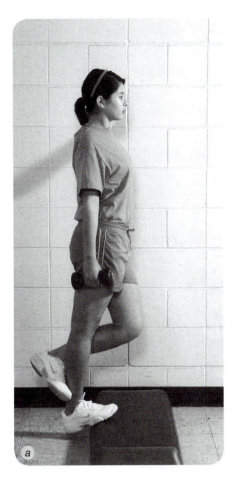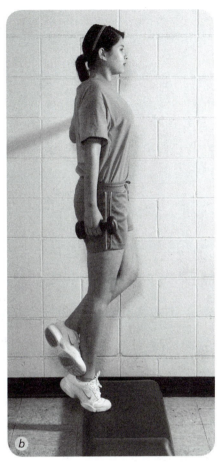

Muscles
Gastrocnemius, soleus

Procedure
1. Begin by grasping a dumbbell in the right hand. Place the ball of the right foot on a board or step with the heel off the surface and leg fully extended. Wrap the left foot behind the right ankle. Use the free left hand for balance by holding on to the wall or bench.
2. Raise up onto the right toe as high as possible; then slowly lower the heel as far as is comfortable. Complete the assigned number of repetitions, and repeat with the opposite leg.

Technique Tip
Concentrate on keeping your torso and knees straight to avoid upper-leg involvement.

TOE RAISE

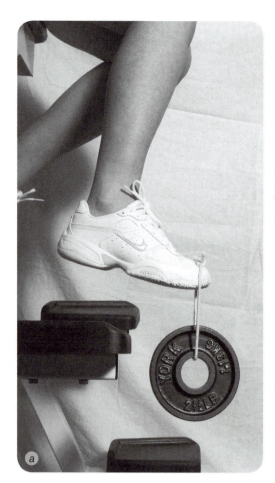 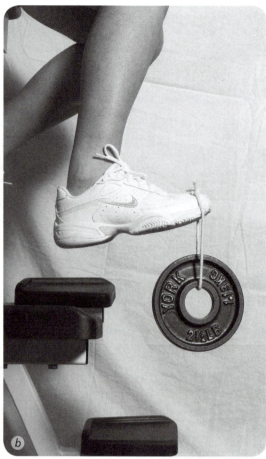

Muscle

Tibialis anterior

Procedure

1. Sit on the edge of a high bench with your legs hanging straight down. Attach one end of a looped rope or elastic band near the toe and ball area of one foot. Attach a light weight to the other end of the rope or band, and let the weight hang freely.
2. Lower the toe and ball of your foot as far as possible.
3. Lift the weight by raising the toe and ball of your foot as high as possible.
4. Pause briefly, then slowly lower the weight to the starting position.

Technique Tips

- You need only a light weight for this exercise because these are small muscles.
- Note that you cannot raise your foot much farther than the horizontal position. Thus, it is important to lower the toe and ball of your foot as much as possible to perform this exercise through the maximum range of motion.

POWER CLEAN

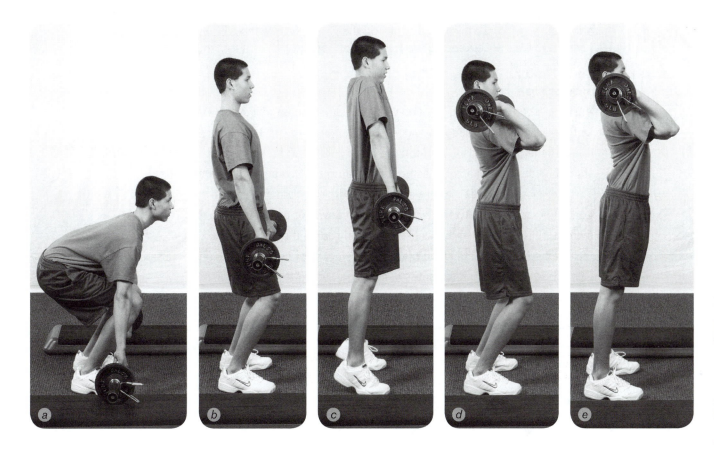

Muscles

Quadriceps, hamstrings, gluteals, gastrocnemius and soleus, erector spinae, latissimus dorsi, upper trapezius, deltoids, biceps

Procedure

1. Begin by standing with feet hip-width apart or slightly wider and toes pointing forward. Squat down and grasp a barbell with an overhand grip slightly wider than shoulder width.

2. Fully extend arms with elbows out to sides. Position barbell over balls of the feet and close to shins. Body weight should be on the midfoot and heel areas.

3. Establish a flat back by pulling shoulder blades together and holding chest up and out.

4. Begin lift by extending the knees. Then move hips forward and raise shoulders at same rate. During this initial movement, keep the angle of the back constant with arms extended. This phase of the lift is performed at a moderate speed.

5. When the barbell is just above the knees, thrust hips forward and continue pulling with elbows extended until the torso is nearly vertical. Rise onto the balls of the feet and shrug the shoulders so the barbell moves upward in a straight path. This rapid movement is similar to a vertical jump.

6. At maximum shoulder elevation, flex and pull with the arms, keeping elbows high.

7. As the barbell approaches the level of the lower chest, rapidly swing both elbows under the barbell. Catch the barbell on the shoulders and upper chest in a one-quarter front squat position with knees slightly bent. Finish the lift by standing tall.

» continued

POWER CLEAN » *continued*

8. Return the barbell to the starting position by popping the barbell off the shoulders with a short dip and press to reduce stress on the wrists. Rotate the elbows and rebend the knees and hips while keeping the torso upright as the bar is caught in the upright position.

Technique Tips

- Assume a correct starting position with the bar of the barbell over the balls of the feet.
- During the initial pull, keep shoulders above or in front of barbell.
- Allow the legs and hips to perform the work during the first phase of this lift.
- Try to pull the barbell as high as possible during the upward movement phase.
- This exercise should be performed in one complete, fluid movement.
- Learn how to perform this lift with a wooden dowel or unloaded barbell.
- Increase the flexibility in the wrists to properly catch the barbell.
- Return the barbell to the lifting platform if you cannot perform the exercise properly.
- Use rubber-coated bumper plates to avoid damaging the floors.
- You can use several variations of this movement to learn the lift properly.

SNATCH

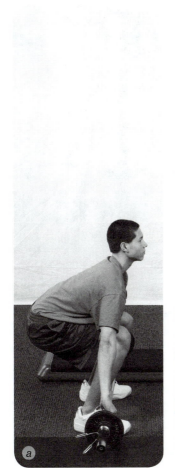
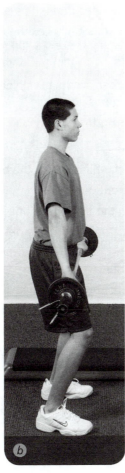
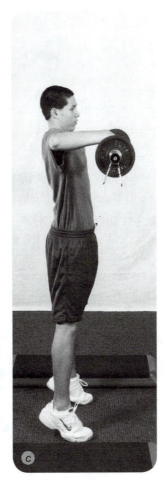
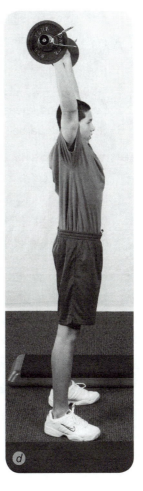

Muscles

Quadriceps, hamstrings, gluteals, gastrocnemius and soleus, erector spinae, latissimus dorsi, upper trapezius, deltoids, biceps

Procedure

1. To determine the correct hand spacing for this exercise, grasp a barbell with an overhand grip. From a standing position, raise the elbows to the side of your body until your elbows reach shoulder height. Move your grip slightly outward until the thumb of each hand is just outside each elbow. While maintaining this grip width, assume the starting position by returning the barbell to the floor. The bar should be just in front of your shins, both arms should be fully extended with elbows out to sides, and feet should be about shoulder-width apart.

2. Establish a flat back by pulling shoulder blades together and holding your chest up and out.

3. Begin lift by extending the knees while keeping shoulders over the barbell. Then move hips forward and raise shoulders at same rate. During this initial movement, keep angle of the back constant with arms extended. This phase of the lift is performed at a moderate speed.

4. When the barbell passes the knees, thrust the hips forward and pull the barbell upward as the torso starts to assume an upright position.

» *continued*

SNATCH » *continued*

5. At full extension, rise up on your toes and shrug your shoulders while pulling the barbell as high as possible. Both elbows should be fully extended during this phase of the lift.

6. As the bar reaches maximum height (about midchest), slightly flex the knees, dropping below the height of the barbell. At the same time, rotate elbows until they are under the barbell.

7. Push with the arms and shoulders to support the barbell overhead with elbows extended. Fully extend knees and hips and assume a standing position.

8. Return the barbell to the starting position by reversing the lifting motion.

Technique Tips

- Assume a correct starting position with the bar of the barbell over the balls of the feet.
- During the initial pull, keep shoulders above or in front of barbell.
- Allow the legs and hips to perform the work during the first phase of this lift.
- As the bar reaches maximum height, bend the knees only enough to get underneath the barbell with elbows fully extended.
- Perform this exercise in one complete, fluid movement.
- Learn how to perform this lift with a wooden dowel or unloaded barbell.
- Return the barbell to the lifting platform if you cannot perform the exercise properly.
- Use rubber-coated bumper plates to avoid damaging the floors.
- You can use several variations of this movement to learn the lift properly.

PUSH PRESS

Muscles

Quadriceps, hamstrings, gluteals, gastrocnemius and soleus, erector spinae, upper trapezius, deltoids

Procedure

1. Begin by grasping a barbell from a rack with an overhand grip slightly wider than shoulder width. The barbell should be supported on the front of the shoulders and upper chest. Stand with feet approximately hip-width apart.

2. Retract head back. Slightly bend the knees, hips, and ankles.

3. Drive the barbell upward by extending the knees and hips and rising up on the toes. When the barbell is slightly higher than the head, rapidly extend both arms to press the barbell to the overhead position.

4. Briefly hold the barbell overhead with arms extended and shoulders in a shrug position.

5. Return the barbell to the starting position in a controlled manner.

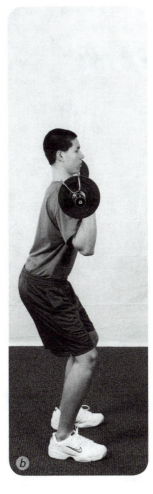 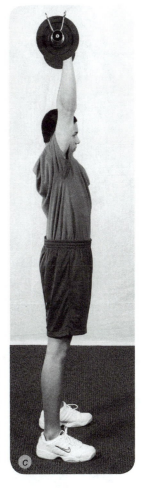

Technique Tips

- Learn how to perform this multijoint lift with a wooden dowel or unloaded barbell.
- Slightly bend the knees and hips when returning the barbell to the starting position.
- Return the barbell to the shoulder position if you cannot complete a repetition.
- Return the barbell to the lifting platform if you lose control of the barbell.
- You can also perform this lift by holding a dumbbell in each hand.

Summary

Strength training with barbells and dumbbells can be safe and effective provided that children are given an opportunity to learn proper exercise technique. Take the time to demonstrate each exercise to all participants and then provide constructive feedback on each child's exercise performance. We encourage children to ask questions and realize that learning free-weight exercises requires coordination and concentration. Unlike some other modes of training, barbells and dumbbells allow unrestrained movement patterns, and therefore children of all sizes can use them in hundreds of exercises. Further, free weights are relatively inexpensive and are readily available at stores that sell sporting goods and fitness equipment.

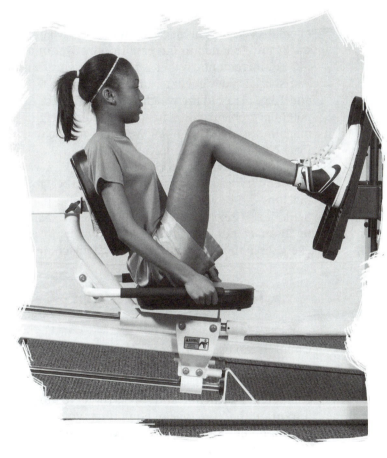

WEIGHT MACHINES

5

The growing interest in strength training for adults and children has led to the development of various types of weight machines, from single-station units to multipurpose machines with 5 to 10 exercise stations. In general, weight machines are easy to use because they provide a fixed movement pattern for each exercise, and most provide support for the body. Because some weight machines allow you to train specific muscle groups, you can also use them to isolate a muscle that is prone to injury. Further, well-designed weight machines attempt to match the weight to your strength by means of a cam or other accommodating resistance device. That is, some machines allow you to maintain a constant level of exertion throughout each repetition. Although weight machines are more expensive than other types of strength-training equipment, they enable you to perform some strength-building exercises that you can't do with free weights, such as the leg curl and front pull-down.

For many years weight machines were made only for adults. Larger teenagers could fit into those machines, but some young weight trainers were too short. Thus, small children could not perform most exercises throughout the full range of motion. Because children's limbs are shorter than those of adults, improper positioning could result in an injury if a child's arm or leg slipped off the pad or if the pad moved during the performance of an exercise. Even though you can easily modify some machines with a few seat pads, such as the shoulder press, you need to account for proper positioning of all body parts and machine-to-body relationships.

Child-sized weight machines are available for young weight trainers.

In all cases, you must do modifications to adult-sized equipment carefully so you never compromise the safety of young lifters. When deciding on equipment needs, realize that children must fit into a weight machine properly in order for the biomechanical requirements of the muscle action to match the training equipment. Above all, if you cannot properly adapt a weight machine to fit the child, do not use that machine. Remember that safety is the most important issue. Generally, you can modify adult machines by adding seat pads beneath the hips or behind the back so the children can perform the exercise in the desired range of motion.

Fortunately, several companies have started to manufacture youth strength-training equipment that is durable, versatile, easy to use, and safe. This type of equipment is similar in design to adult-sized machines, but it is scaled down to fit smaller bodies. Single-station units and multistation machines that use pin-operated weight stacks or weight plates are available. One great advantage of child-sized weight machines is that the weight stacks are designed to increase in only 5-pound (~2 kg) increments. If that is too heavy, you can add specially designed 1- and 2.5-pound (~0.5 and 1 kg) plates to the weight stack as needed. A potential problem with some types of adult weight machines is that the initial weight is too heavy for a child, or the 10- to 20-pound (~5 to 9 kg) increases in weight are too large. Although there are many types of adult- and child-sized weight machines, the structure and function of a particular exercise, such as the leg press, is the same on all machines. Thus, you can easily adapt the exercises in this chapter to your weight machines.

Training on Weight Machines

Children can use most types of strength-training equipment safely and effectively, provided that they follow appropriate guidelines. Caring and competent instruction and supervision are more important than the type of equipment you have in your home or at your school. If you have access to adult-sized weight machines, make the necessary modifications to ensure proper fit. Remember that, in many cases, simply adjusting the seat height does not necessarily mean that a child can safely fit onto a piece of equipment. No matter what type of weight machines you use—adult or child size—take the following safety steps before and during your exercise sessions:

- Check for frayed cables, worn chains, and loose pads.

- Carry all weight plates with two hands.
- Adjust seats and pads as needed.
- Insert the selector pin all the way into the weight stack.
- Keep hands away from chains, belts, pulleys, and cams.
- Never place your hands or feet between the weight stacks.
- Concentrate on lifting and lowering the weights under control. Do not drop the weight to the starting position.
- Teach correct breathing techniques (exhale during the lifting phase and inhale during the lowering phase).

Caring and competent instruction and supervision are more important than the type of equipment you have in your home or at your school. If you have access to adult-sized weight machines, make the necessary modifications to ensure proper fit.

Weight Machine Exercises

The weight machine exercises in this chapter are organized into two major sections: lower body and upper body. Included are the names of the primary muscles strengthened by each exercise. This format should make it easy for teachers and coaches to choose exercises that train all the major muscle groups. Remember that it is important to create balance in your strength-training workout so that you exercise opposing muscle groups equally. For example, if you perform a chest exercise, you should also perform an exercise for your upper back. Make sure participants feel the exercise effort in the target muscle groups, as indicated in the exercise descriptions.

Create balance in your strength-training workout so that you exercise opposing muscle groups equally.

LEG PRESS

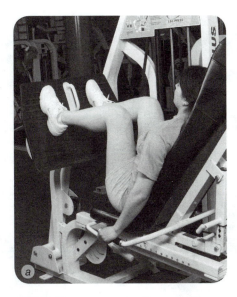
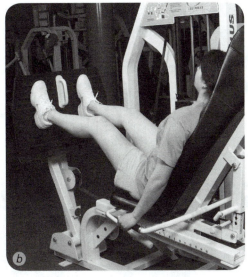

Muscles

Quadriceps, gluteals, hamstrings

Procedure

1. Adjust the back pad so that you flex your knees to 90 degrees.

2. Sit with your back firmly against the back pad. Place your feet on the footpad, in line with your knees and hips. Grip the handles to keep your buttocks on the seat throughout the exercise.

3. Press evenly with both feet until you almost extend, but don't lock, your knees.

4. Return to starting position by slowly bending your knees. Then begin the forward movement before the weight touches the stack.

Technique Tips

- Do not lock your knees in the extended position.
- Keep both feet flat on the footpad throughout the full movement.
- Keep your back pressed against the seat.
- Keep hands away from moving parts.

Child-Sized Equipment

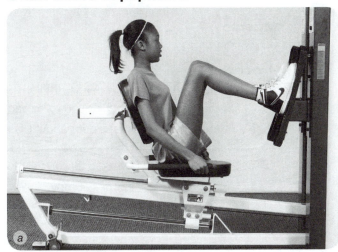

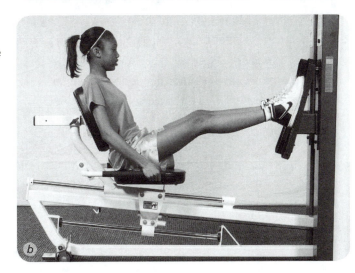

LEG EXTENSION

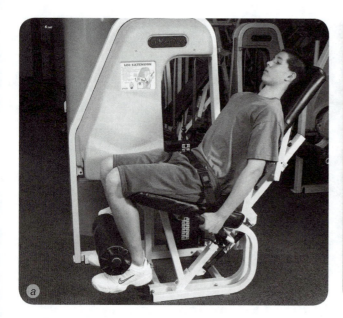
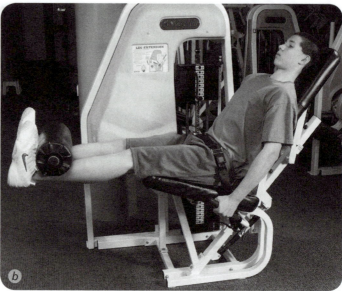

Muscle

Quadriceps

Procedure

1. Adjust the back pad so that your knees are in line with the machine's axis of rotation. Position your ankles behind the roller pad.
2. Sit erect with your knees bent about 90 degrees and your back firmly against the pad. Grip both handles.
3. Lift the roller pad upward until you fully extend your knees.
4. Return to the starting position by slowly bending your knees. Then begin the upward movement before the weight touches the stack.

Technique Tips

- Grip the handles firmly to keep your buttocks on the seat throughout the exercise.
- Do not drop weight quickly to starting position.
- Upper body should not move during exercise.
- Adjust ankle pad to child's length.
- Grasp handles throughout exercise.

LEG CURL

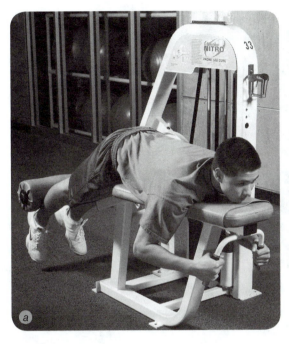
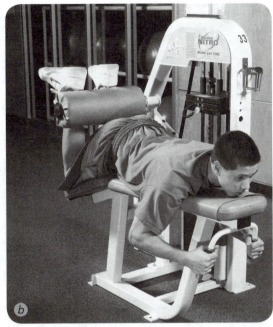

Muscle
Hamstrings

Procedure

1. Adjust the roller pad so that your knees are in line with the machine's axis of rotation. Position your lower legs under the roller pad.
2. Lie face down with your legs extended and your knees just off the bench. Grip both handles.
3. Pull the roller pad toward your hips until your knees are bent beyond 90 degrees.
4. Return slowly to starting position and repeat.

Technique Tips

- Keep your chest and chin in contact with the bench during this exercise.
- Learn this exercise with a light weight at first.
- Grasp handles throughout the exercise.
- Keep head in line with the body at all times.

HIP ADDUCTION

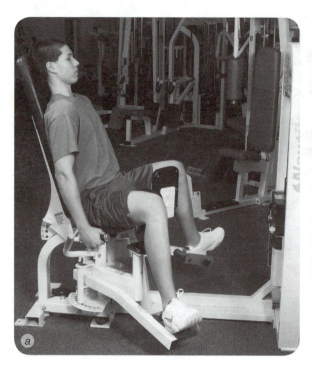
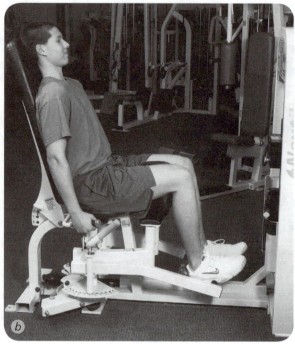

Muscle

Hip adductor

Procedure

1. Sit on the machine with your shoulders and back against the pad. Place your legs on the rungs of the machine with your ankles on the supports.
2. Adjust the movement lever to an appropriate starting position with the legs apart. Grasp the handles.
3. Slowly squeeze your legs together as far as possible; return to starting position.

Technique Tips

- Do not begin this exercise from an overstretched position.
- You can also perform this exercise on a standing hip adduction machine. Face the machine and adjust the pad to just above knee level.

HIP ABDUCTION

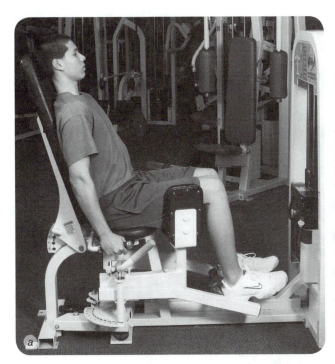 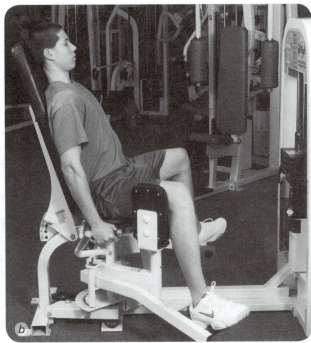

Muscle

Hip abductor

Procedure

1. Sit on the machine with your shoulders and back against the pad. Place your legs on the rungs of the machine with your ankles on the supports.

2. Slowly pull your legs apart as far as possible; return to starting position.

Technique Tips

- Grip the handles to keep buttocks in contact with the seat.
- You can also perform this exercise on a standing hip abduction machine. Face the machine and adjust the pad to just above knee level.

HEEL RAISE

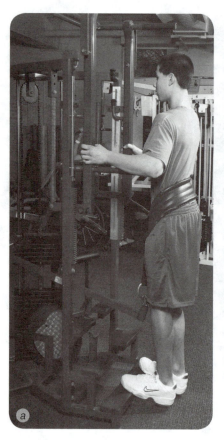 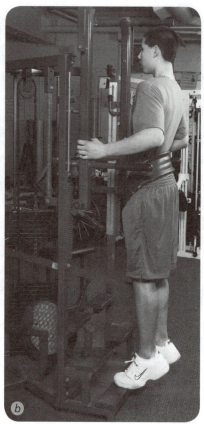

Muscles

Gastrocnemius, soleus

Procedure

1. Place the belt securely around your waist; then stand with the balls of both feet on the edge of the step. Place your hands on the bar for support.

2. Slowly lift your heels as high as possible while keeping your knees straight. Then return to the starting position, lowering your heels below step level.

Technique Tips

- Wear appropriate footwear when performing this exercise.
- Maintain an erect posture with knees straight during this exercise.
- Do not bounce out of the bottom position.

CHEST PRESS

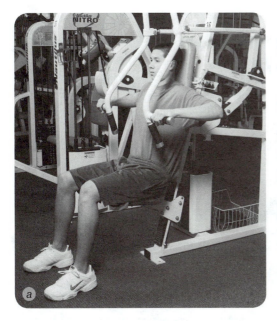
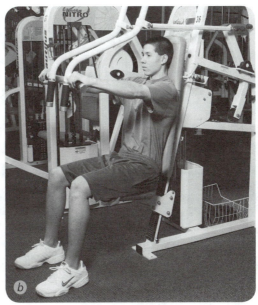

Muscles

Pectoralis major, anterior deltoid, triceps

Procedure

1. Position yourself so the handles are at chest level. Grasp the handles.

2. Keep your head, shoulders, and back on the bench.

3. Push the handles upward until you have almost extended, but not locked, your arms. Keep your wrists straight.

4. Slowly return the handles to the starting position. Then begin the movement before the weight touches the stack.

Technique Tips

- Do not lock your elbows in the extended position.
- Do not arch or twist your back when performing this exercise.

Child-Sized Equipment

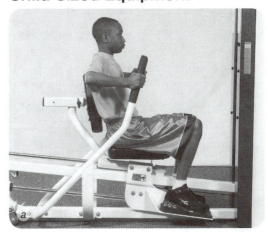

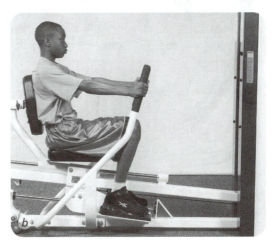

SEATED ROW

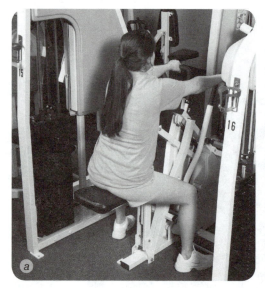

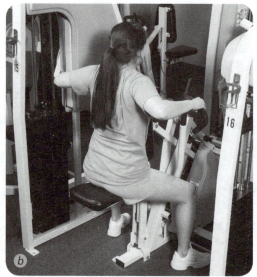

Muscles

Latissimus dorsi, biceps

Procedure

1. Adjust the seat so the handles are at shoulder level. Sit with your chest against the pad, torso erect, and feet on the floor. Grasp both handles.

2. Pull the handles back toward the side of your chest, keeping your chest on the pad.

3. Slowly return the handles to the starting position. Then begin the movement before the weight touches the stack.

Technique Tips

- Pause at the chest, then slowly return to the starting position.

- Do not twist your back or allow your chest to come off the pad when performing this exercise.

Child-Sized Equipment

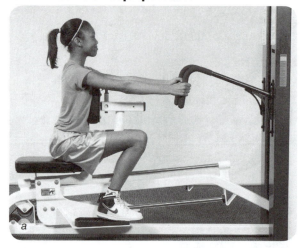

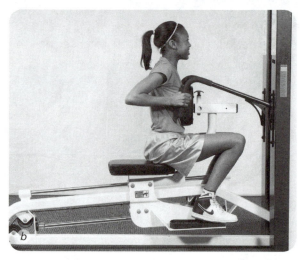

FRONT PULL-DOWN

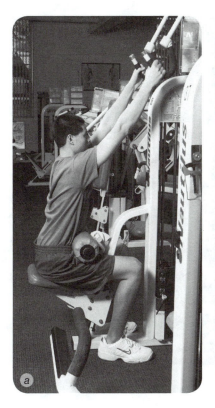
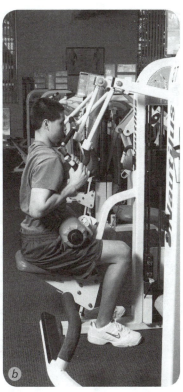

Muscles

Latissimus dorsi, biceps

Procedure

1. Grip the bar underhand (palms toward your face), about shoulder-width apart.

2. Sit on the seat, placing both knees under the restraining pads and keeping your upper torso erect and arms straight.

3. Slowly pull the bar downward below your chin. Then allow the bar to return slowly until you fully extend your arms.

Technique Tips

• Do not twist your torso when performing this exercise. Use only your arms and upper back to complete the exercise

• Keep the bar and cable away from your face during this exercise.

Child-Sized Equipment

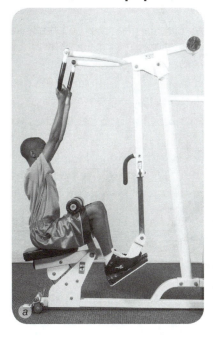
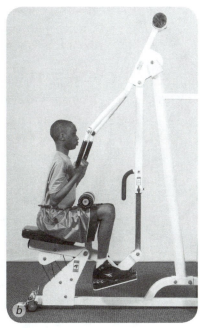

PULLOVER

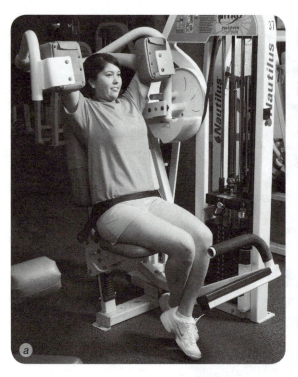 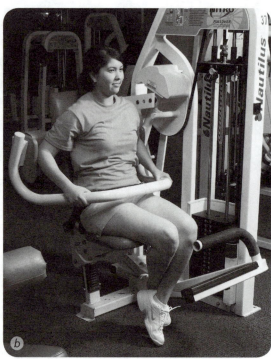

Muscle

Latissimus dorsi

Procedure

1. Sit with your back against the pad, seat belt firmly secured, and shoulders in line with the machine's axis of rotation. Press the foot lever forward and bring the arm pads into position.

2. Position your elbows on the pads and place both hands on the bar. Slowly release the footpad, and allow your feet to hang in front of your body.

3. Pull the arm pads downward until the bar touches your waist. Slowly return to starting position and repeat.

4. When finished, place your feet on the footpad, and press forward to hold the weight stack. Remove your arms and slowly lower the weight stack using feet or legs.

Technique Tips

• Keep your hands open and elbows against the pad during this exercise.

• Return weight to starting position at a controlled speed.

• Keep back pressed firmly against the seat.

OVERHEAD PRESS

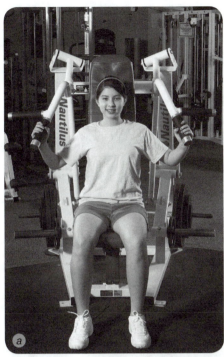

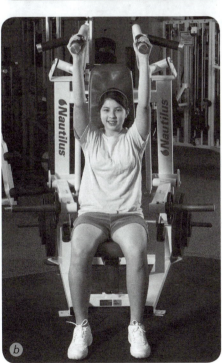

Muscles
Deltoids, upper trapezius, triceps

Procedure
1. Adjust the seat so the handles are directly in front of the shoulders.
2. Sit with your back against the pad and torso erect.
3. Grasp the handles with a palms-forward grip about shoulder-width apart.
4. Slowly push both arms overhead until you almost fully extend, but don't lock, your elbows.
5. Slowly return to the starting position. Then begin the movement before the weight touches the stack.

Technique Tips
- Keep your torso erect during this exercise.
- Learn this exercise with a relatively light weight load.

Child-Sized Equipment

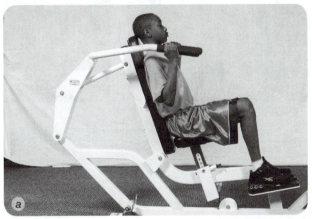

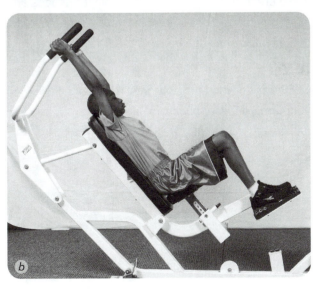

LATERAL RAISE

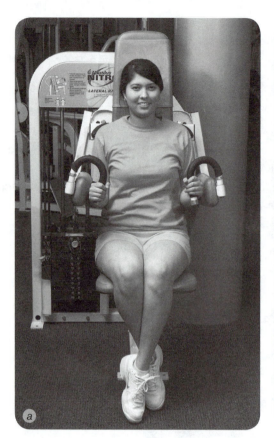
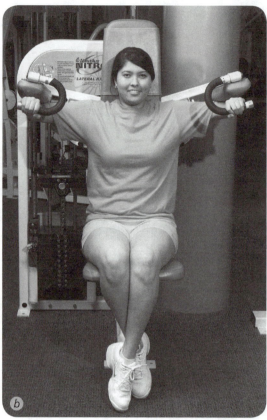

Muscle
Deltoids

Procedure

1. Adjust the seat so the center of the shoulders is in line with the axes of rotation. Sit with your torso erect, and place your arms against the pads and your hands on the handles.
2. Slowly lift both arms upward, keeping your wrists straight.
3. Stop when your arms are parallel to the floor. Return to starting position.

Technique Tips

- Do not lift arms beyond the horizontal position.
- Use your arms, not your hands, for lifting.

TRICEPS EXTENSION

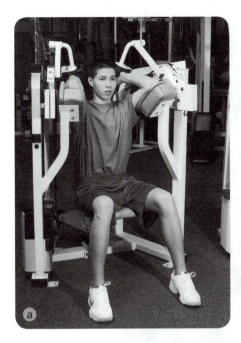

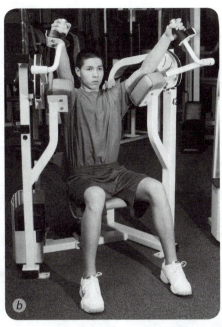

Muscle

Triceps

Procedure

1. Adjust the seat so both elbows are in line with the machine's axis of rotation.
2. Sit with your back against the pad, torso erect, and feet on the floor.
3. Place sides of hands against hand pads and allow pads to move close to shoulders.
4. Slowly push both hand pads forward until you fully extend your arms. Then return to the starting position, beginning the movement before the weight touches the stack.

Technique Tips

- Keep your upper arm on the pads during the forward and backward movements.
- Keep your wrists straight during this exercise.

Child-Sized Equipment

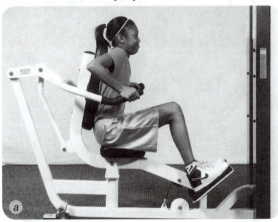

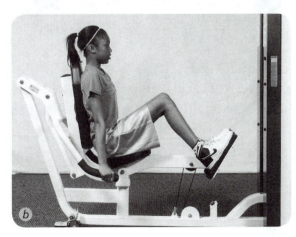

TRICEPS PRESS-DOWN

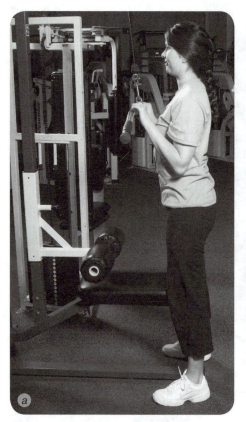 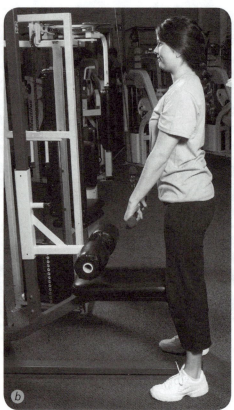

Muscle

Triceps

Procedure

1. Stand in front of the lat bar with your torso erect and knees slightly bent.
2. Grasp the bar with both hands in an overhand grip (palms facing the floor) and your hands shoulder-width apart.
3. Begin with the bar at the upper chest and your upper arms against your sides.
4. Slowly press your forearms downward until you fully extend your arms.
5. Slowly return to the starting position, beginning the movement before the weight touches the stack.

Technique Tips

- Keep your torso erect, and do not allow your elbows to move forward or bow outward.
- You can attach a short bar or other training accessories to the cable for this exercise.

BICEPS CURL

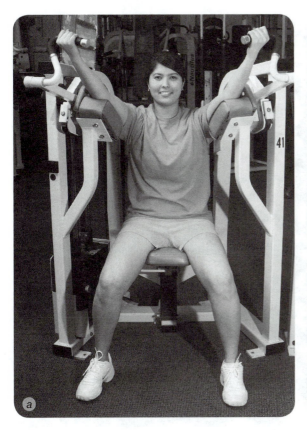 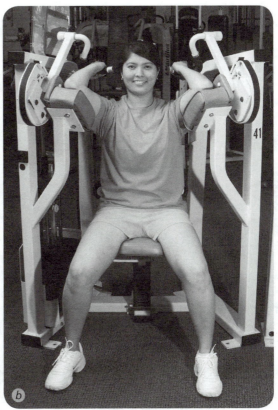

Muscle
Biceps

Procedure
1. Adjust the seat so both elbows are in line with the machine's axis of rotation.
2. Sit with your chest against the pad, torso erect, and feet on the floor.
3. Grasp the handles with an underhand grip, elbows slightly bent.
4. Slowly curl the handles upward until you fully flex your arms. Then return to the starting position, beginning the movement before the weight touches the stack.

Technique Tips
• Keep your upper arms on the pads and your wrists straight during this exercise.
• When finished, stand to remove your hands from the machine.

ABDOMINAL CURL

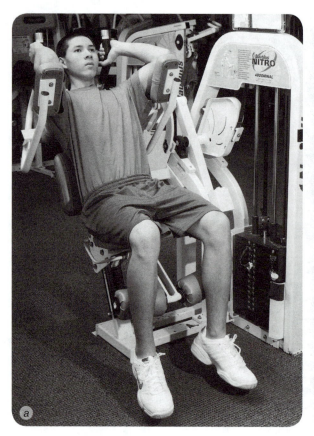
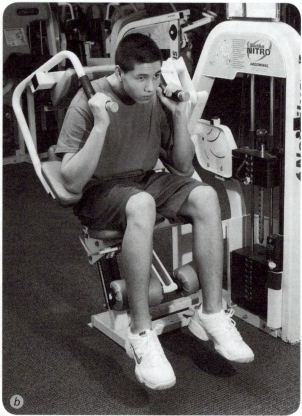

Muscle

Rectus abdominis

Procedure

1. Adjust the seat so your navel is aligned with the machine's axis of rotation. Chest pads should be at chest level.
2. Sit with your back against the pad, elbows on the pads, hands on the grips, and feet relaxed.
3. Slowly curl your torso forward until you fully flex your trunk. Then return to the starting position, beginning the movement before the weight touches the stack.

Technique Tips

- Shorten the distance between the rib cage and the navel by contracting the abdominal muscles. Do not use your hands and shoulders.
- Avoid fast and jerky movements during this exercise.

LOWER-BACK EXTENSION

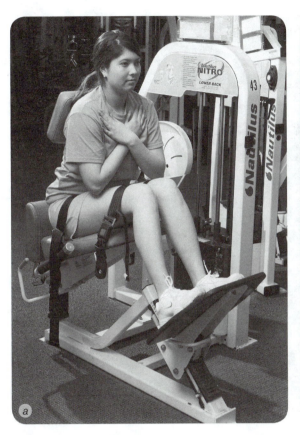 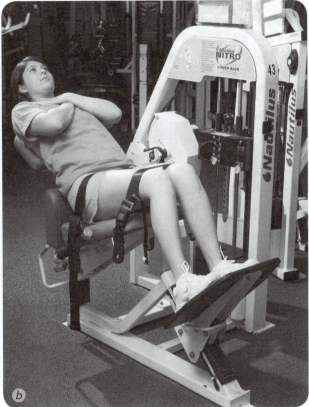

Muscle

Erector spinae

Procedure

1. Adjust the seat so the navel is aligned with the machine's axis of rotation.
2. Sit with your back against the pad, arms folded across your chest, and feet firmly placed on the footpad.
3. Slowly extend your torso backward until you reach full trunk extension.

Technique Tips

- Do not allow the upper body to freefall during the downward phase of this exercise.
- Avoid fast and jerky movements during this exercise.

ROTARY TORSO

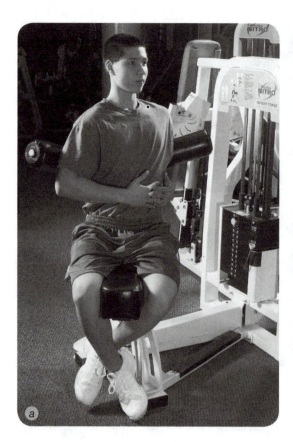

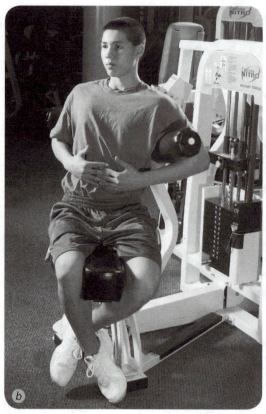

Muscles

Rectus abdominis, external obliques, internal obliques

Procedure

1. Sit on the machine, facing forward with your legs around the seat extension.
2. Place your left arm behind and your right arm against the movement pads.
3. Slowly turn your torso to the right and pause briefly. Return to the starting position.
4. Perform the desired number of repetitions; then change the seat position and arm positions and repeat to the left side.

Technique Tips

- Rotate your torso as far as possible, but stay within a pain-free range of motion.
- Breathe continuously while performing this exercise.

NECK FLEXION

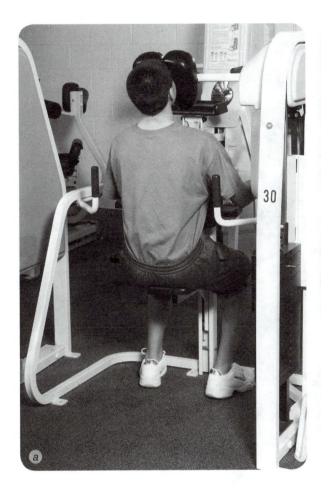
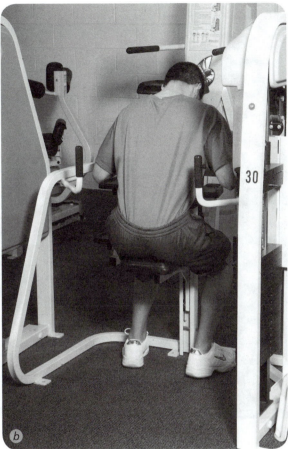

Muscle

Neck flexor

Procedure

1. Adjust the seat and chest pad to the appropriate positions. Your face should fit in the face pad and your body should be erect.

2. Place your forehead and cheeks against the face pad with your head angled slightly backward. Grasp the handles.

3. Slowly push your head forward until your neck is comfortably flexed. Return to the starting position.

Technique Tips

- Maintain chest contact with the pad during the exercise, and avoid fast or jerky movements.
- Breathe continuously while performing this exercise.

NECK EXTENSION

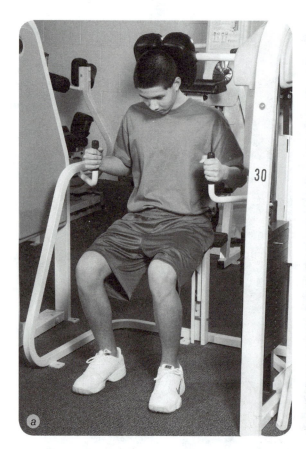
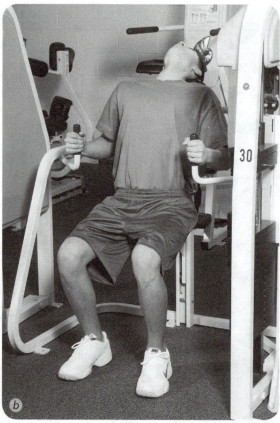

Muscle

Neck extensor

Procedure

1. Adjust the seat and torso pad to the appropriate positions. The back of your head should fit in the head pad.
2. Place the back of your head against the head pad with your head angled slightly forward. Grasp the handles.
3. Slowly push your head backward until your neck is comfortably extended. Return to the starting position.

Technique Tips

- Maintain back contact with the pad during the exercise, and avoid fast or jerky movements.
- Breathe continuously while performing this exercise.

SUPER FOREARM

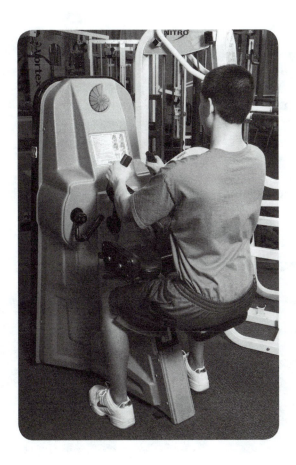

Muscles
Wrist flexor, wrist extensor, wrist supinator, wrist pronator, finger gripper

Procedure
This machine provides five separate exercises for the various muscles of the forearms. A qualified instructor should demonstrate each movement properly.

Technique Tips
- Keep torso erect throughout each exercise.
- Keep forearms on restraining pads throughout each exercise.

ROTARY SHOULDER

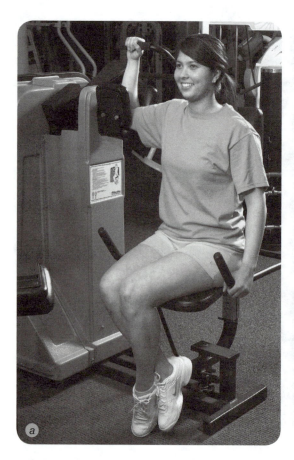
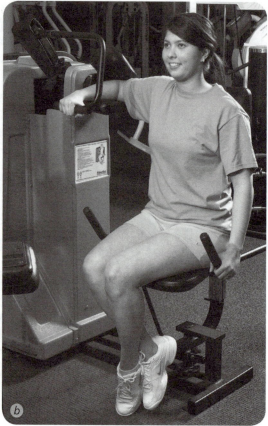

Muscles

Shoulder rotator cuff, teres minor, infraspinatus, supraspinatus, subscapularis

Procedure

This machine provides four separate exercises for the internal and external rotator muscles of the shoulder. A qualified instructor should demonstrate each movement properly.

Technique Tips

- Keep torso erect throughout each exercise.
- Keep elbow firmly secured in restraining cuff throughout each exercise.
- Use relatively light weight for the weaker internal rotation movements.

Summary

Weight machines are durable, versatile, safe, and easy to use. Although most teenagers fit into weight machines designed for adults, several companies manufacture child-sized equipment that accommodates the smaller bodies of preadolescents. In either case, participants must fit into weight machines properly for safe and productive training. Also, it is important to remind participants to keep their hands and feet away from moving chains, pulleys, and weight stacks. With proper instruction and supervision, children and teenagers can easily learn how to use various types of weight machines that train all of the major muscle groups. Machine training provides support, structure, and specific movement patterns that facilitate the learning process for a safe and effective exercise experience.

ELASTIC BANDS AND MEDICINE BALLS

6

Elastic bands and medicine balls are safe and effective alternatives to free weights and machines. Bands and balls not only are inexpensive and fun to use but also add variety to a child's workout routine. Elastic bands and medicine balls come in various shapes and sizes, so children can start at safe levels and progress as needed. Some elastic bands look like rubber cords with handles at each end, whereas other types are made from strips of 6-inch-wide (15 cm) elastic material. We use medicine balls and elastic bands in our youth fitness classes because several children can exercise simultaneously, and they can perform many exercises. Further, children don't normally need spotting when performing exercises with medicine balls and elastic bands, provided that they have appropriate guidance and instruction.

Strength training with an elastic band involves performing exercises with the force required to stretch the elastic material and return it to its unstretched state. Commercial rubber cord products are available from sporting good and fitness equipment stores, or you can make bands from a length of elastic material. You can perform exercises for the upper and lower body by either holding the ends of the band with your hands or attaching the elastic band to a fixed object. As children get stronger, you can increase the resistance by adjusting the amount of prestretch on the band or by using a thicker band that will provide additional resistance. However, when performing exercises with an elastic band, note

that the resistance is greatest as the movement nears completion, which is different from other modes of strength training. Thus, it is important to use an elastic band that allows smooth execution of the exercise through the full range of motion.

Medicine balls are made of weighted vinyl, polyurethane, or leather and are available in various sizes. Some medicine balls have a textured surface or a handle for easier gripping, and others are inflatable and bounce. Adult athletes have used medicine ball exercises for many years, and now more children are benefiting from this mode of training. Unlike the traditional methods of strength training, medicine ball exercises condition the body through dynamic movements that you can perform either slowly or rapidly. Because you typically perform exercises on machines and free weights at a moderate speed (due to the nature of the equipment and the weight used), fast-speed medicine ball training can add a new dimension to a child's workout program. In that regard, some youth are very strong but are not very powerful (strong and quick) because they have not trained their muscles to contract quickly. Training with medicine balls can enhance the body's neuromuscular adaptations to strength training since some medicine ball exercises require explosive speed and high power outputs.

By using medicine balls of varied weights and sizes, you can develop a conditioning program consisting of throwing and catching movements

99

for the upper body, rotational exercises for the trunk, and extension exercises for the lower body. Most notably, you can use medicine balls to strengthen the core of a child's body, which is central to all movements. The core includes the abdominals as well as the hip and lower-back musculature. We have found that medicine ball training is a challenging, motivating, and worthwhile method of developing strength, speed, power, and coordination in children of all ages and abilities. In our programs we use color-coded balls and elastic bands so the instructors and the children can easily keep track of the loads they are using.

Although commercially made medicine balls are relatively inexpensive and are readily available from most sporting good and athletic equipment companies, you can make your own medicine balls for a fraction of the cost of what you would pay a retailer. Homemade medicine balls are durable and can be used for numerous exercises, but they do not bounce very well, and you should not stand or sit on them for balance training. Water-filled volleyballs weigh about 6 to 8 pounds (2.7 to 3.6 kg); if sand is used in place of water, the ball is heavier. Since the weight of these balls is too heavy for most beginners, we use smaller playground balls to make 2- to 4-pound (1 to 2 kg) medicine balls for children. Most of our homemade balls have lasted for over a year, and even if they start to leak, water does little or no damage to most athletic surfaces and the leak can easily be repaired. The steps in the sidebar show you how to make your own medicine balls.

HOW TO MAKE A MEDICINE BALL

Step 1. You can use an old soccer ball, a volleyball, a basketball, or even a small rubber playground ball. Using a pair of long-nose pliers, carefully insert the open prongs in and around the plug, then gently grasp the plug with the pliers. Slowly pull the plug out with a slight rocking motion; be careful not to rip the ball. Once the plug is removed, save it to be reinserted later.

Step 2. Fill the ball with water or sand, depending on how heavy you want to make the ball. To fill the ball, use a small funnel or a piece of wax paper rolled into the shape of a funnel. Insert the end of the funnel into the ball. If you fill it with water, use a fine stream from a faucet or watering can. Periodically squeeze the air out of the ball.

Step 3. When the ball is full of water, squeeze some plumber's glue onto the plug and into the hole, then reinsert the plug. The ball should be ready to use in a few hours.

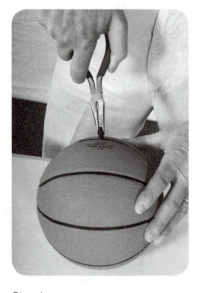 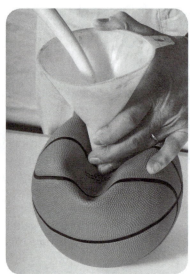 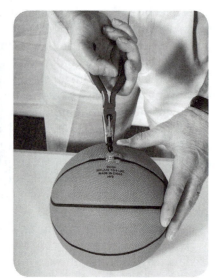

Step 1.   Step 2.   Step 3.

Training With Elastic Bands and Medicine Balls

Before you use bands or balls, check that they are not torn or have abnormal spots of wear and tear. Do not use elastic bands that are torn or frayed for any exercise, because the cord could snap and cause an injury. Although most medicine balls can last for years, check the balls to be sure they are well constructed. Leather balls should be professionally stitched, and vinyl and polyurethane balls should be properly inflated. Again, it is worth emphasizing that elastic bands and medicine balls can be safe and effective for children, if adults provide competent instruction and supervision. Although elastic bands and medicine balls may seem harmless, they are not toys. Do not allow horseplay in the training area, and remind children that they can get hurt if they use the equipment improperly.

Strength-training exercises that use elastic bands and medicine balls often require more skill and coordination than weight machines because children need to create and control the movement pattern. Therefore, adults need to provide clear instructions, and children should begin with a lightweight medicine ball or a thin rubber cord. Also note that the amount of stretch on the band at the start of the exercise will affect the amount of resistance the child feels. When a child performs elastic band exercises, adjust the child's hand position on the cord so he or she begins each exercise with an appropriate amount of stretch. In some cases it might be necessary to grasp a section of the tubing rather than the handles themselves. Depending on body size, limb length, and baseline strength level, a child's hand position on the band will vary. Discourage breath holding and teach youth how to breathe correctly when training with elastic bands and medicine balls.

> Strength-training exercises that use elastic bands and medicine balls often require more skill and coordination than weight machines because children need to create and control the movement pattern.

Elastic Band Exercises

You can use the elastic band exercises to strengthen the upper and lower body. Remember that training with a resistance band requires more skill and coordination than some other types of strength-training equipment. Beginning with a thin band and focusing on the correct technique will give children an opportunity to learn how to stabilize their bodies when their arms or legs are working against the resistance of an elastic cord. Note that the resistance from the bands will be greatest when the exercise motion nears completion. That is, unlike other types of strength-building equipment, the exercise will become more difficult at the end. Remind boys and girls that it is important to maintain proper form throughout the full range of motion.

> Beginning with a thin band and focusing on the correct technique will give children an opportunity to learn how to stabilize their bodies when their arms or legs are working against the resistance of an elastic cord.

ELASTIC BAND SQUAT

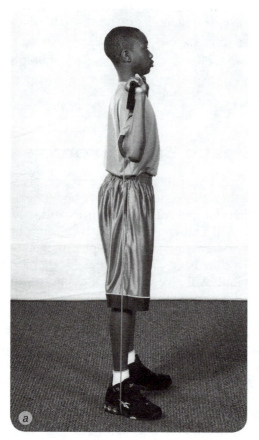
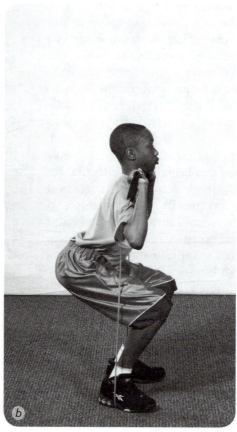

Muscles

Quadriceps, gluteals, hamstrings

Procedure

1. Begin by grasping the ends of an elastic band in each hand, and stand erect with both feet on top of the middle of the cord to hold it stationary.

2. Raise your hands to shoulder level with palms facing forward. The band should be behind your shoulders.

3. Slowly bend your ankles, knees, and hips until your thighs are parallel to the floor. Keep your back flat, head up, and eyes fixed straight ahead.

4. Return to starting position by slowly straightening your knees and hips.

Technique Tips

• Your knees should follow a slightly outward pattern of the feet. Do not let the knees cave in.

• Avoid bouncing out of the bottom position.

• Concentrate on keeping your head up and chest out. Avoid excessive forward lean.

ELASTIC BAND LEG CURL

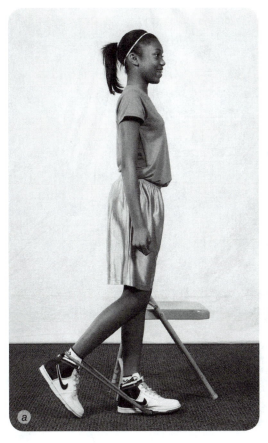
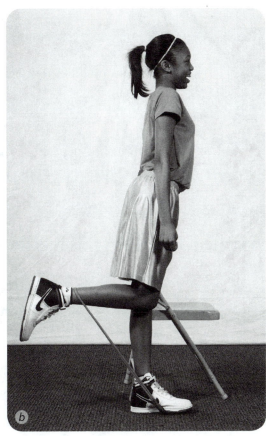

Muscle

Hamstrings

Procedure

1. Put one handle of the cord through the opening near the other handle to create a small loop.

2. Put your right foot inside the loop and place the band behind your right ankle. Stand on the rubber cord with your left foot.

3. Slowly curl your right leg backward toward your buttocks while maintaining an erect posture. Return your leg to the starting position, and perform the desired number of repetitions. Repeat on the other side.

Technique Tips

- Keep the nonexercising leg stationary during this exercise.
- Use a thin band at first.
- If necessary, place one hand on a wall or chair for balance.

ELASTIC BAND STANDING CHEST PRESS

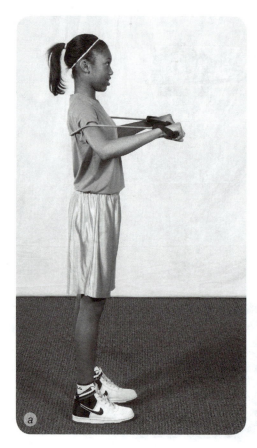
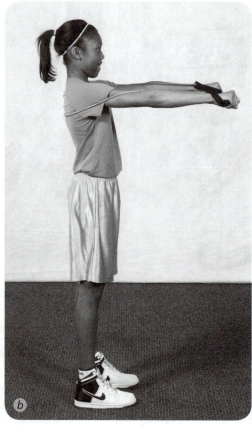

Muscles
Pectoralis major, anterior deltoid, triceps

Procedure
1. Stand with your feet about shoulder-width apart and the resistance band wrapped around the back of your shoulders.
2. Grasp the ends of the cord firmly, and place both hands (palms facing the floor) in front of your shoulders with your elbows flexed.
3. Slowly straighten your elbows until you fully extend both arms. Then return to the starting position and repeat.

Technique Tips
- Do not twist or arch your body.
- Extend both arms at an even rate.

ELASTIC BAND SEATED SHOULDER PRESS

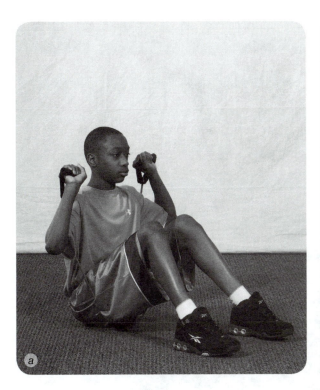
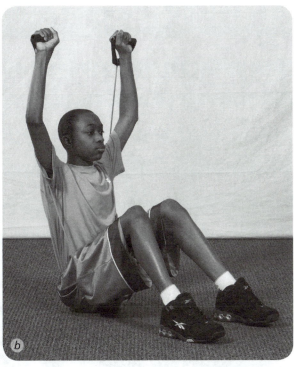

Muscles

Deltoids, upper trapezius, triceps

Procedure

1. Begin by sitting on the floor on the middle of a resistance band while holding one end of the band in each hand.
2. Hold the band at shoulder height with your palms facing away from your body.
3. Slowly push both arms upward until you fully extend them over the shoulders. Then lower your arms to the starting position and repeat.

Technique Tips

- Sit erect and keep your lower back straight by contracting your abdominal and lower-back muscles.
- Extend both elbows completely over shoulders.

ELASTIC BAND UPRIGHT ROW

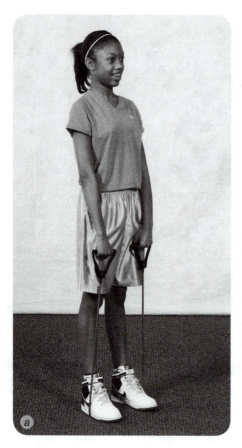 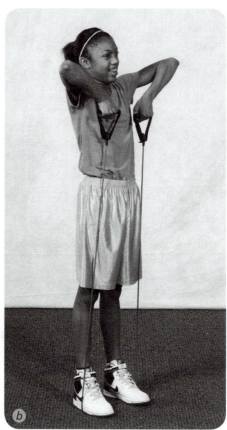

Muscles

Deltoids, upper trapezius, biceps

Procedure

1. Begin by grasping one end of the band in each hand with palms facing your body; stand erect with both feet on top of the cord about hip-width apart. Hold the band so that it hangs straight down in front of your body with your hands closer than shoulder-width apart.

2. Slowly pull the band along the abdomen and chest toward the chin while keeping both elbows pointing out to the sides; then lower the cord to the starting position.

Technique Tips

- Stand erect and keep the cord close to your body during this exercise.
- At the top of the movement the elbows should be slightly higher than the shoulders.

ELASTIC BAND LATERAL RAISE

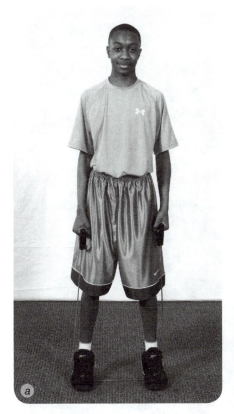
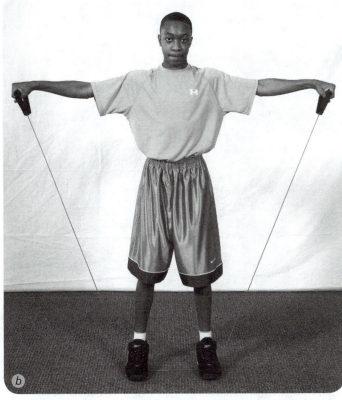

Muscle
Deltoids

Procedure
1. Begin by grasping one end of the band in each hand and standing erect with both feet on top of the band about hip-width apart. Hold the band so that it hangs straight down at your sides with your palms facing your body and elbows slightly bent.
2. Slowly lift both arms upward and sideward until your arms are level with your shoulders (arms parallel to floor). Keep elbows slightly bent and return to starting position.

Technique Tips
* Stand erect and keep your lower back straight by contracting your abdominal and lower-back muscles.
* Don't raise your arms higher than parallel to the floor.

ELASTIC BAND LAT PULL-DOWN

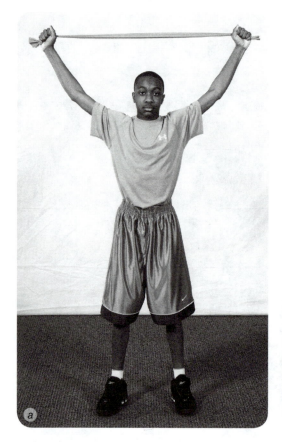
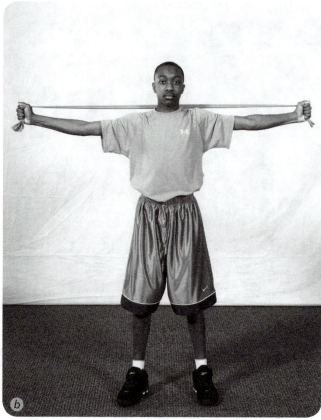

Muscles

Latissimus dorsi, biceps

Procedure

1. Grip a section of the band with your hands about shoulder-width apart, and fully extend your arms overhead. Stand erect with your hands wider than your shoulders and your palms facing forward.

2. Slowly pull your arms downward until the band is behind your neck and your arms are parallel to the floor. Then return slowly to starting position.

Technique Tips

- Use only your arms and upper back to complete the exercise. Focus on pulling your shoulder blades together and keeping your arms in line with your body.

- Fold the band in half for greater resistance.

ELASTIC BAND SEATED ROW

Muscles
Latissimus dorsi, biceps

Procedure
1. Begin by wrapping the band around your feet. Grasp the handles of the cord. Sit on the floor with your knees slightly bent, your back straight, and your palms facing each other.

2. Pull the band handles back toward the sides of your body; then slowly return the handles to the starting position.

Technique Tips
- Be sure the resistance band is securely wrapped around your feet. Point your toes forward slightly to prevent the band from slipping off your feet.

- As an alternative, place the resistance band around an immovable object while in the seated position.

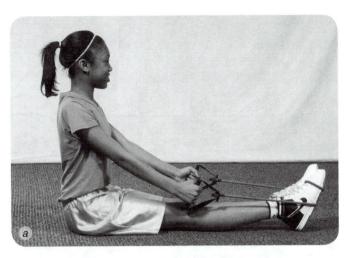

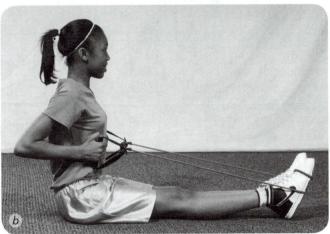

ELASTIC BAND BICEPS CURL

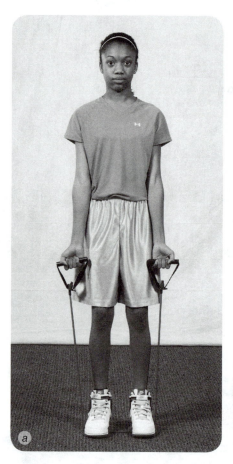
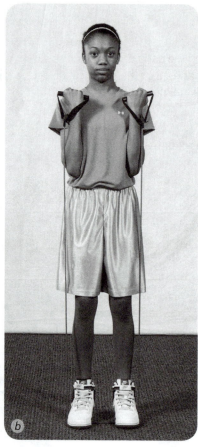

Muscle
Biceps

Procedure

1. Begin by standing on top of the band with your body erect and both hands grasping the band handles. Place your feet about hip-width apart, and fully extend your arms with your palms facing forward and arms at your sides.

2. Slowly curl both hands upward toward your shoulders until your palms face the chest. Then lower both arms to the starting position.

Technique Tips

- Stand erect and keep your lower back straight by contracting your abdominal and lower-back muscles.

- If necessary, stand with your back against the wall to prevent upper-body movement.

- Do not step off the band unless your arms are in the starting position.

ELASTIC BAND TRICEPS EXTENSION

Muscle

Triceps

Procedure

1. Begin by sitting on the middle of a resistance band while holding one end of the band in each hand.

2. Place both hands behind your head with your palms facing the ceiling. The elbows should be bent.

3. Slowly push one arm upward until you fully extend it over your head. Then lower your arm to the starting position, and repeat with your other arm.

Technique Tips

• Only the elbow and forearm should move during this exercise.

• Be sure you secure the band beneath your buttocks.

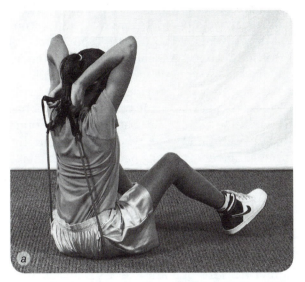

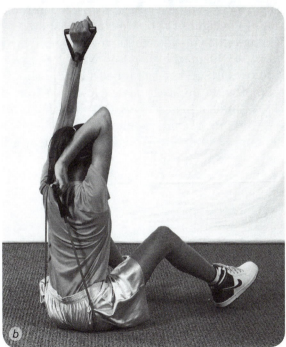

Medicine Ball Exercises

You can control the intensity of a medicine ball exercise by the weight of the medicine ball and the speed at which you perform the exercise. While seasoned adult athletes often use medicine balls that weigh over 11 pounds (5 kg), in our youth programs we begin with 2-pound (1-kg) medicine balls and gradually progress as strength and exercise technique improve. Once children have mastered the proper form, we gradually increase the speed of some exercise movements, the weight of the medicine ball (by about 1 pound [0.5 kg] at a time), and, when appropriate, the distance between training partners. By gradually increasing the speed of movement and the weight of the ball, you can use this type of training to enhance the strength and speed of muscle action.

It is desirable to have medicine balls of various weights and sizes on hand to accommodate the needs and abilities of all children. You will need lighter balls for one-arm exercises and heavier balls for two-arm exercises. Also, keep in mind that the weight of the medicine ball should be less than the weight a child would typically use on a weight machine or free-weight exercise. Additionally, all medicine ball training should take place in an area that is clean and free of clutter and has high ceilings. Overcrowded gymnasiums increase the likelihood that a child will get hurt or bump into a piece of equipment. All participants must follow safety guidelines (e.g., shoes tied and no gum chewing) and exercise directions (e.g., look at training partner and keep hands in ready position). Medicine balls should be securely stored on a rack or in a bin when they are not in use.

The medicine ball exercises are organized into three sections: warm-up, strength, and power exercises. The specific muscles used are listed for the strength exercises, whereas the power exercises list general body parts. Just as for other modes of training, you should perform warm-up and strength exercises with medicine balls at a moderate speed and in a controlled manner; you should perform power exercises at a faster speed provided that you maintain proper form. Before performing power exercises, always do a few warm-up repetitions of the same exercise at a slower speed. In our program, children perform the power exercises with medicine balls before strength exercises, because if they are fatigued before performing the power exercises they will have difficulty generating near-maximal power, which is the goal of the exercise.

Before performing power exercises, always do a few warm-up repetitions of the same exercise at a slower speed.

The following five exercises are warm-ups for the entire body and therefore specific muscle groups are not mentioned.

AROUND THE WORLD

Procedure

1. Stand with your feet about shoulder-width apart, and hold a light medicine ball over your head with your knees slightly bent and your arms fully extended.

2. Move the ball in a giant circle, bending your knees as the ball moves to the bottom of the circle and straightening your knees as the ball moves to the top of the circle. Complete the desired number of repetitions; then move the ball in the opposite direction.

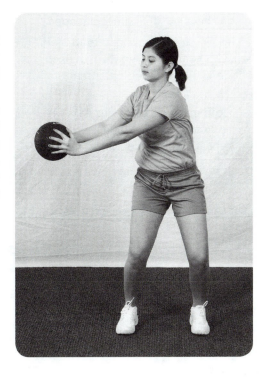

WOOD CHOPPER

Procedure

1. Stand with your feet shoulder-width apart and hold a medicine ball over your head with your knees slightly bent and your arms extended.

2. Bend at the waist and knees while swinging the ball down between legs in a chopping action. Return to the starting position and repeat for the desired number of repetitions.

3. For variety, perform a diagonal chop by starting with the ball overhead and behind the right ear and swinging the ball diagonally across the body to the outside of the left knee. Then repeat on opposite side. Allow feet to rotate to allow for a greater range of motion.

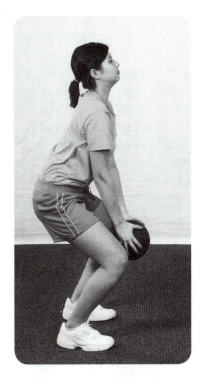

RUSSIAN TWIST

Procedure

1. Stand with your feet shoulder-width apart and hold a medicine ball in front of your waist with knees slightly bent and your arms extended.

2. Alternate twisting to the right and to the left for the desired number of repetitions. Allow feet to rotate to allow for a greater range of motion.

3. For variety, perform a single-leg Russian twist by doing this exercise while standing on one foot. Then repeat on opposite foot.

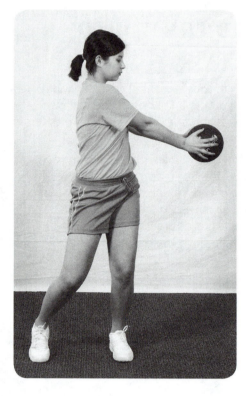

KNEE LIFT

Procedure

1. Stand with your feet about shoulder-width apart, and hold a light medicine ball in front of your body at chest height.

2. As you lift one knee to waist level, touch the ball to the knee; then return the ball and knee to starting position. Repeat with opposite leg.

3. For variety, pass ball under knee as you lift knee to waist level. Then return to the starting position and repeat with opposite leg.

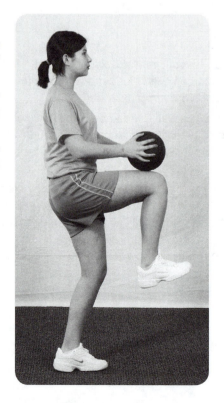

JOG AND CATCH

Procedure

1. Stand with your feet about shoulder-width apart, and hold a light medicine ball in front of your body at waist height.

2. Jog in place while tossing the ball in the air and catching it. Children can clap their hands while the ball is in the air or they can toss the ball to a partner.

3. For variety, jog in place while pressing the ball overhead, tossing ball to right and left hands or moving the ball around your body.

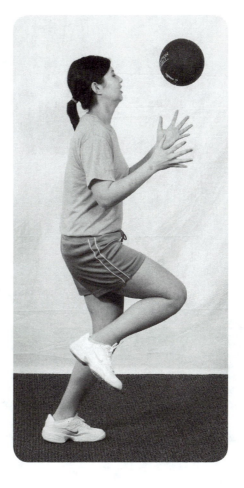

MEDICINE BALL FRONT SQUAT

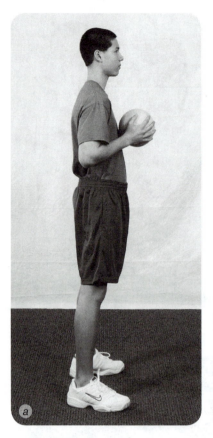
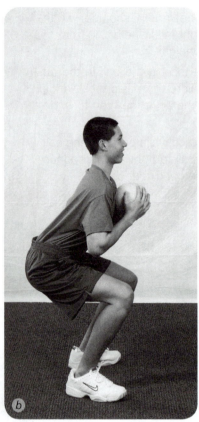

Muscles

Quadriceps, gluteals, hamstrings

Procedure

1. Begin by holding a medicine ball directly in front of your chest with your feet about hip-width apart and toes pointing slightly outward.
2. Slowly bend your ankles, knees, and hips until your thighs are parallel to the floor. Keep your back flat, head up, and eyes fixed straight ahead.
3. Return to the starting position by slowly straightening your knees and hips.

Technique Tips

* Your knees should follow a slightly outward pattern of the feet. Do not let the knees cave in.
* Avoid bouncing out of the bottom position.
* Concentrate on keeping your head up and chest out. Avoid excessive forward lean.
* For variety, perform an overhead squat by holding a medicine ball overhead with your arms fully extended. Follow procedures as noted previously, keeping your arms extended during the exercise and the ball directly over your head.

MEDICINE BALL SINGLE-LEG DIP

Muscles

Quadriceps, gluteals, hamstrings

Procedure

1. Stand on the right foot and hold a medicine ball directly in front of your body.

2. Slowly bend your right ankles, knees, and hips a few inches, keeping your right knee behind your right toes.

3. Keep your back flat, head up, and eyes fixed straight ahead.

4. Return to the starting position and repeat for the desired number of repetitions. Repeat on opposite side.

Technique Tips

- Dip only about 4 inches (10 cm).

- Concentrate on keeping your head up and chest out. Avoid excessive forward lean.

- This exercise can be performed without a ball or with one hand on a wall for balance.

- To perform a single-leg dip and reach, place a medicine ball on the floor about 2 or 3 feet (0.6 to 1 m) from your body. As you bend your left leg, reach with your right hand to touch the ball. Return to the starting position and repeat for the desired number of repetitions. Then repeat on opposite side.

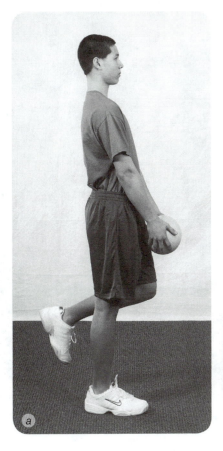

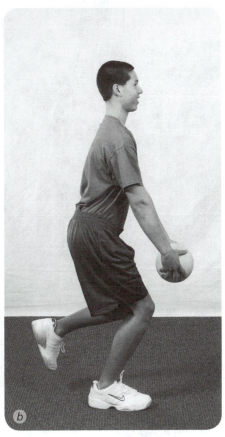

Single-Leg Dip and Reach

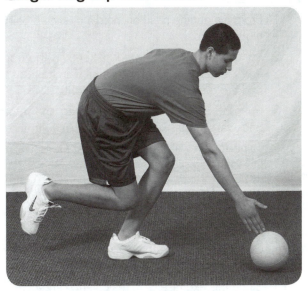

MEDICINE BALL LUNGE

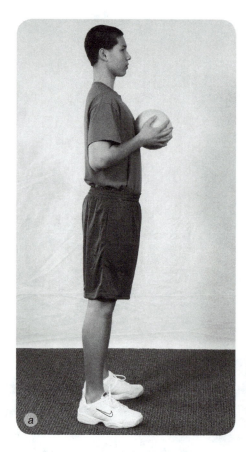
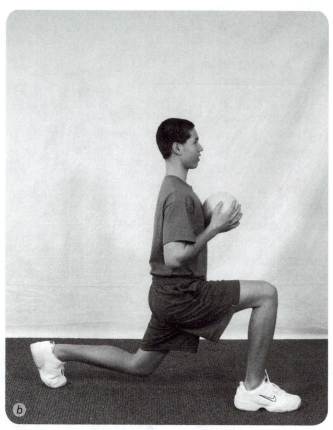

Muscles

Quadriceps, gluteals, hamstrings

Procedure

1. From a standing position, hold a medicine ball in front of your waist with your feet about hip-width apart.

2. Lunge forward with right leg, keeping the front knee behind the toes of the front foot and the ball in front of the chest. The knee of the rear leg should almost touch the floor and the torso should remain upright.

3. Push off the floor with the front leg and return to the starting position with two short backward steps. Repeat the exercise with the opposite leg.

4. To perform a walking lunge, repeat the forward action by alternating legs without returning to the starting position.

Technique Tips

• The lunge should be long enough so that the knee of the front leg does not go in front of the toes.

• Concentrate on keeping your chest out and eyes fixed straight ahead. Avoid excessive forward lean.

• Since this exercise requires balance and coordination, begin with a lightweight medicine ball.

MEDICINE BALL FRONT SHOULDER RAISE

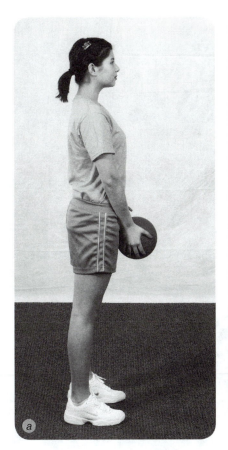

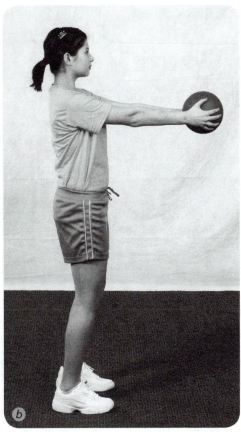

Muscle

Deltoids

Procedure

1. Begin by holding a medicine ball in front of your waist with both hands. Stand erect with your feet about hip-width apart.
2. Slowly lift the ball upward until your arms are at shoulder height; then return to the starting position and repeat.

Technique Tips

- Stand erect and keep your lower back straight by contracting your abdominal and lower-back muscles.
- Don't raise your arms higher than parallel to the floor.

MEDICINE BALL SUPINE CHEST PRESS

Muscles

Pectoralis major, anterior deltoid, triceps

Procedure

1. Lie on a flat bench holding a medicine ball on your chest.

2. Slowly press the ball off your chest until you fully extend both arms. Then slowly return to starting position.

Technique Tips

- Keep the ball above your chest, not above your face.

- Pause briefly in the bottom position before pressing up to complete the movement.

- If a flat bench is not available, lie on the floor to perform this exercise

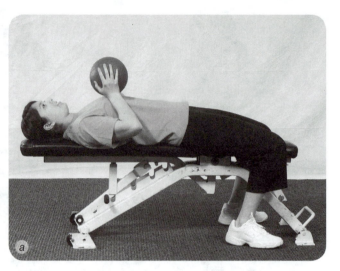

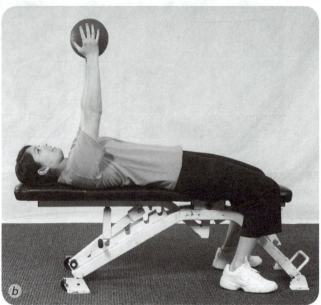

MEDICINE BALL PUSH-UP

Muscles

Pectoralis major, anterior deltoid, triceps

Procedure

1. Start in the push-up position with one hand on the floor and one hand on a regular-sized medicine ball (about the size of a volleyball).

2. Lower your chest until your elbows are at 90 degrees and then return to the starting position.

3. Perform the desired number of repetitions and then repeat with the ball under the other hand.

Technique Tips

- Maintain a flat back throughout the exercise.

- You can perform this exercise in a modified position with both knees on a mat.

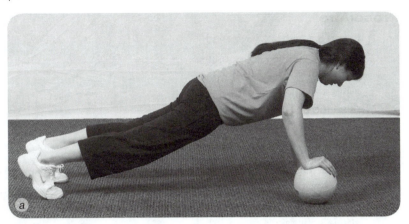

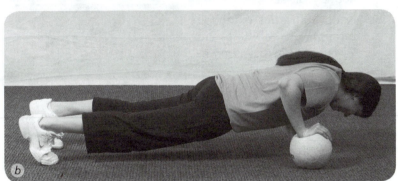

MEDICINE BALL PULLOVER

Muscle

Latissimus dorsi

Procedure

1. Lie on a bench holding a medicine ball behind your head with both arms extended.
2. While keeping arms extended, raise the ball over chest area. Return to starting position and repeat.

Technique Tips

- In the ending position, keep the ball above your chest, not above your face.
- Keep both arms extended throughout the lifting and lowering phases of this movement.

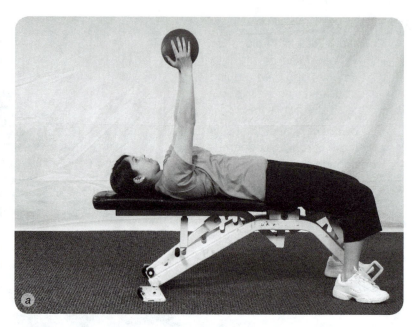

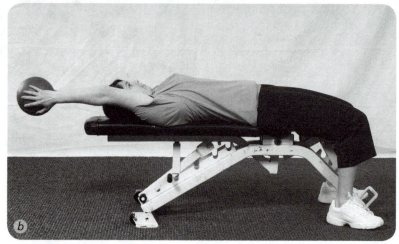

MEDICINE BALL TRICEPS PRESS

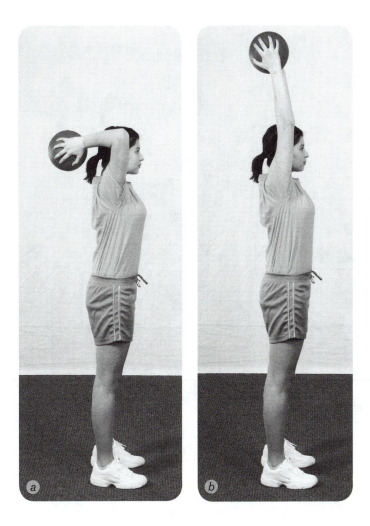

Muscle
Triceps

Procedure
1. Stand erect with your feet about hip-width apart. Hold a medicine ball behind your head with your elbows flexed at ear level.
2. Press the ball overhead until you fully extend your arms. Then slowly return to starting position and repeat.

Technique Tips
- Stand erect and keep your lower back straight by contracting your abdominal and lower-back muscles.
- Only the elbows and forearms should move during this exercise.

MEDICINE BALL BICEPS CURL

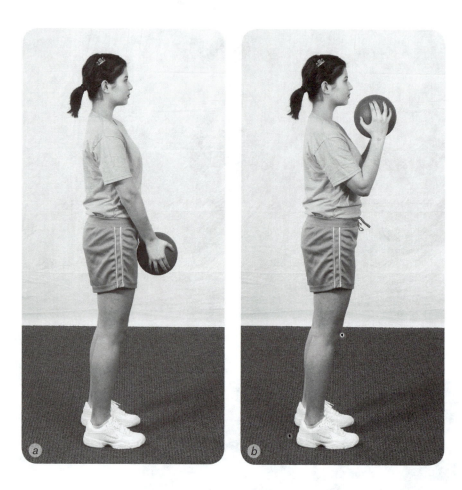

Muscle

Biceps

Procedure

1. Stand erect with your feet about hip-width apart. Hold a medicine ball in front of your waist with your arms fully extended.

2. Curl the ball toward your face, keeping your back straight. Then slowly return to starting position and repeat.

Technique Tips

• Stand erect and keep your lower back straight by contracting your abdominal and lower-back muscles.

• Only the elbows and forearms should move during this exercise.

MEDICINE BALL CURL-UP

Muscle

Rectus abdominis

Procedure

1. From a curl-up position on the floor with knees bent at 90 degrees, hold a ball against your chest with both hands.

2. As you curl forward lifting shoulder blades off the mat, extend both arms and touch knees with ball. Return to starting position and repeat for the desired number of repetitions.

Technique Tips

- Keep your lower back in contact with the mat during this exercise.

- For variety, begin with both legs extended toward the ceiling. Curl upward, lifting shoulder blades off the mat while pressing ball toward feet.

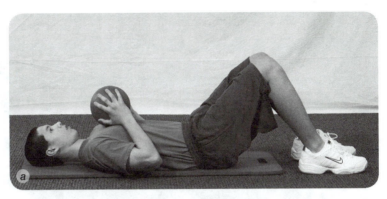

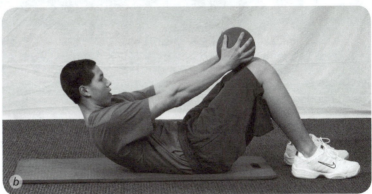

MEDICINE BALL TWO-HAND HOLD

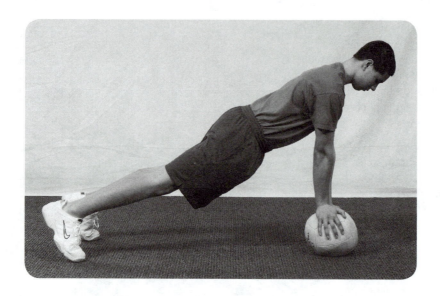

Muscles

Rectus abdominis, pectoralis major, deltoids, triceps

Procedure

1. From a push-up position, place both hands on a leather ball while keeping arms extended, back flat, and feet shoulder-width apart.
2. Hold this position for the desired amount of time (e.g., 10 to 30 seconds), then relax.

Technique Tips

- Breathe normally when performing this exercise.
- For variety, maintain the desired position while lifting one hand off the ball or one foot off the floor.

MEDICINE BALL TWIST AND TURN

Muscles

Rectus abdominis, internal oblique, external oblique

Procedure

1. Sit on the floor with your knees bent at a 45-degree angle and your feet on the floor. Hold a medicine ball in front of your chest.

2. Rotate your upper body from side to side, touching the floor with the ball on each side.

Technique Tips

- Lean back slightly while rotating your body from side to side.

- For variety, perform a partner twist by having two children sit or stand back to back. They pass the ball to each other in a circle for a desired number of repetitions and then change the direction.

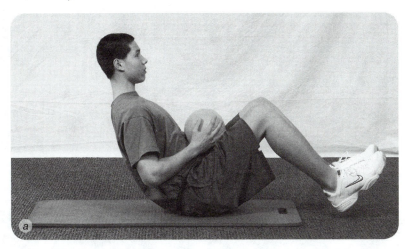

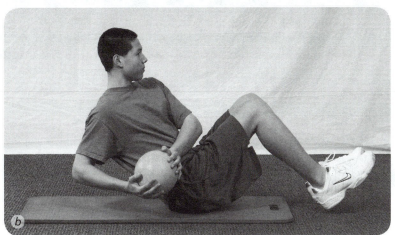

MEDICINE BALL LOWER-BACK PULL

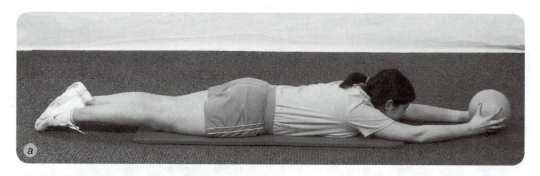

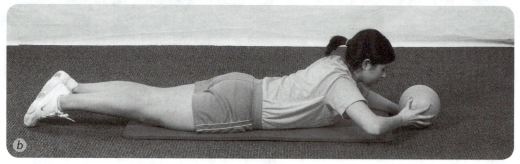

Muscle

Erector spinae

Procedure

1. Lie facedown on a mat with arms and legs extended while holding a ball with both hands outstretched.
2. Pull ball toward body as you lift your chest off the floor and then press out and return to the starting position.

Technique Tips

- Lift your chest only a few inches off the floor.
- Breathe normally when performing this exercise.

MEDICINE BALL SQUAT TOSS

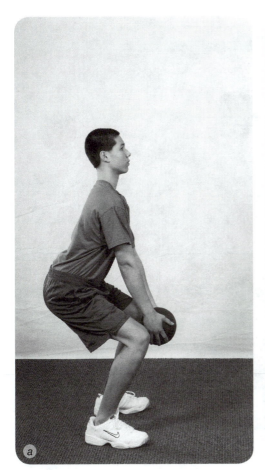
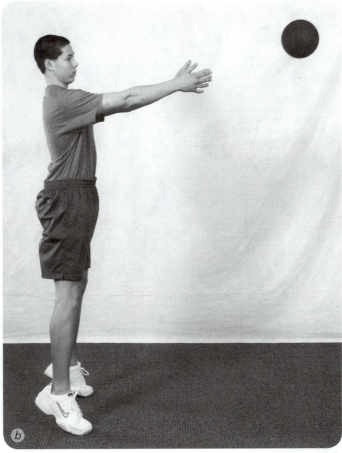

Muscles

Legs, chest, shoulders, arms

Procedure

1. Begin by holding a medicine ball directly in front of your body with your feet about hip-width apart and toes pointing slightly outward.
2. Bend your ankles, knees, and hips until your thighs are parallel to the floor. Keep your back flat, head up, and eyes fixed straight ahead.
3. Quickly jump upward and toss the ball as high as you can in front of you.

Technique Tips

- On the downward motion, your knees should follow a slightly outward pattern of the feet. Do not let the knees cave in.
- Avoid bouncing out of the bottom position.

MEDICINE BALL LUNGE PASS

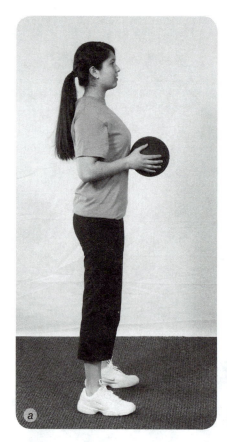
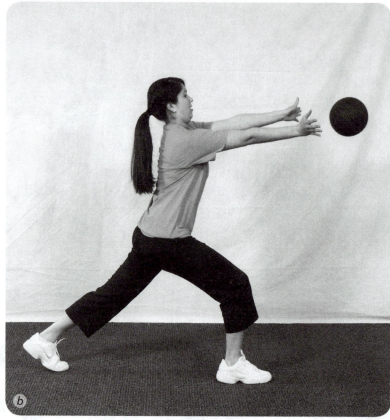

Muscles

Legs, chest, shoulders, arms

Procedure

1. Begin by holding a medicine ball in front of your chest with feet about hip-width apart.
2. Take a long step forward, and quickly push the ball off your chest.

Technique Tips

- Keep your upper torso erect after you release the ball. Do not lean forward.
- Step far enough in front of your body so that your front knee is bent to nearly 90 degrees.

MEDICINE BALL CHEST PASS

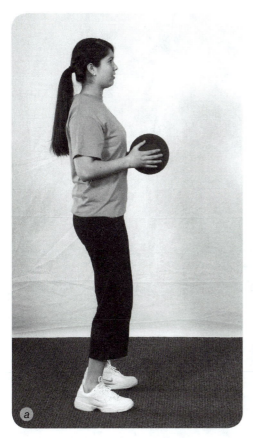

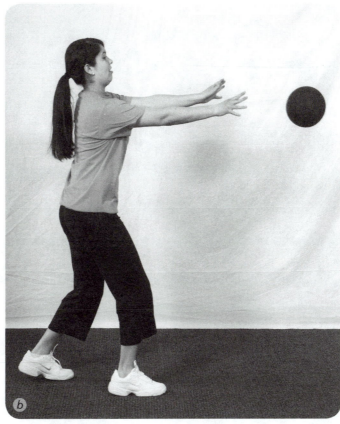

Muscles

Chest, shoulders, arms

Procedure

1. Stand erect while holding a medicine ball at chest level with both hands.
2. Step forward and quickly press the ball off your chest.

Technique Tips

- Keep your upper torso erect after you release the ball. Do not lean forward.
- A partner can stand about 10 feet away and catch the ball after one bounce. Over time the distance between partners can increase. The greater the distance, the greater the effort that is required.
- For variety, perform this exercise while kneeling or sitting on the floor. Keep your body straight as you push the ball off your chest.

MEDICINE BALL SIDE PASS

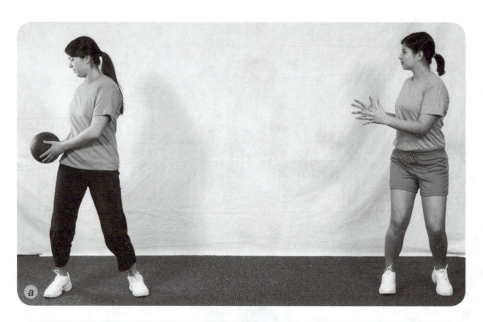

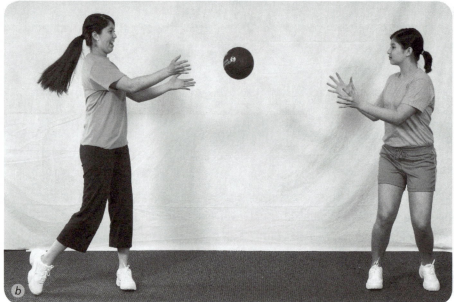

Muscles
Trunk, arms

Procedure
Stand with your side facing your partner. With the ball at about waist level, swing it across your body and pass it to your partner. When you have performed the desired number of repetitions, stand with the other side of your body facing your partner and repeat.

Technique Tips
- Release the ball with more weight on front foot.
- Rotate back foot to allow for a greater range of motion.

MEDICINE BALL PUSH

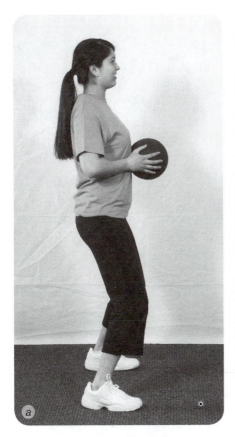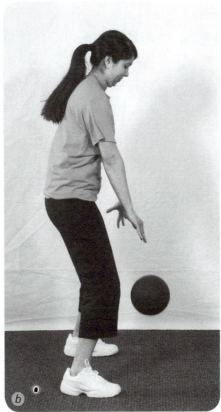

Muscles

Chest, shoulders, arms

Procedure

1. Stand with feet shoulder-width apart and knees slightly bent. Hold a medicine ball against the chest with both hands.
2. Push the ball downward as fast as possible and release toward the floor.
3. Catch the ball after one bounce and repeat.

Technique Tips

- Use chest, shoulder, and arm muscles to push the ball toward the floor.
- Use a rubber medicine ball for this exercise.

MEDICINE BALL OVERHEAD THROW

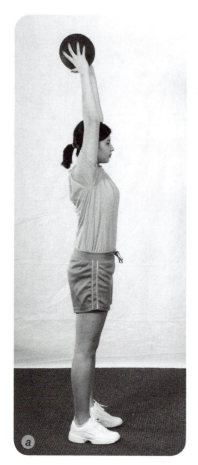
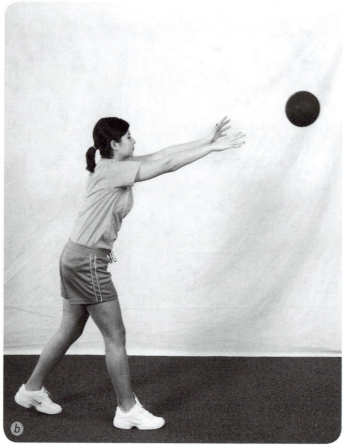

Muscles

Legs, shoulders, trunk, arms

Procedure

1. Hold the medicine ball overhead with arms bent.
2. Step forward and throw the ball as far forward as possible.
3. A partner should catch the ball after one bounce and repeat the exercise.

Technique Tips

- Use legs, shoulder, trunk, and arm muscles to throw the ball.
- Throw the ball against a wall if a partner is not available.
- Use a rubber medicine ball for this exercise.

MEDICINE BALL BACKWARD THROW

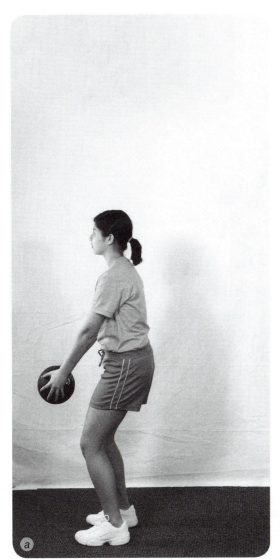
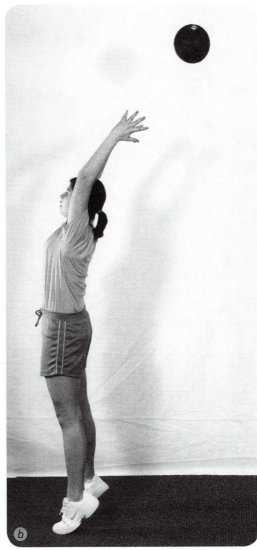

Muscles

Legs, shoulders, trunk, arms

Procedure

1. Stand and hold a medicine ball in front of the body with arms extended.
2. Lower body slightly while keeping arms straight.
3. Quickly rise up and throw the ball over your head as far backward as possible.

Technique Tips

- Extend your ankles, knees, and hips as you throw the ball over your head.
- Always make sure the area behind you is clear before you throw the ball. Partners should not attempt to catch the ball.

MEDICINE BALL SINGLE-ARM TOSS

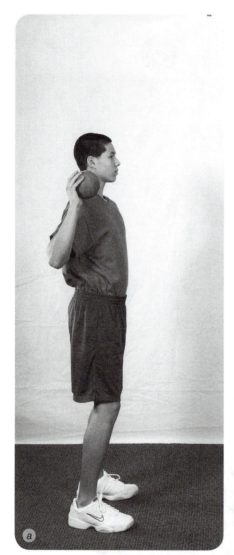
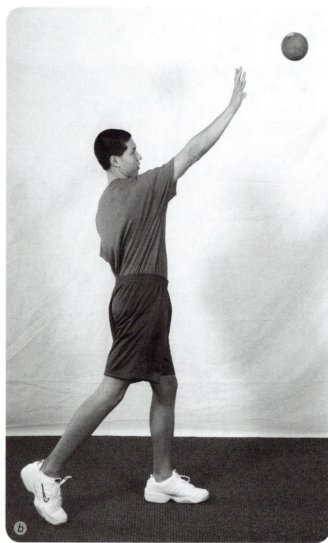

Muscles

Trunk, shoulders, arms

Procedure

1. Hold a small medicine ball in the right hand at ear level.
2. Step forward with the left foot and toss the ball as far forward as possible. Repeat with your other side.

Technique Tips

- Because this is a single-arm exercise, begin with a lightweight medicine ball and gradually progress as you get stronger.
- For variety, perform this exercise while kneeling on the floor.

Summary

Elastic bands and medicine balls are inexpensive and fun to use, and they can add a new dimension to a child's workout routine. Adults have used elastic bands and medicine balls for many years, and now these pieces of equipment are available in a variety of shapes and sizes that are appropriate for children. Children and teenagers of all sizes and abilities can perform numerous exercises with medicine balls and elastic bands to enhance strength, power, balance, and coordination. Since strength training with elastic bands and medicine balls involves skill and coordination, take time to provide clear instructions and begin with a thin elastic band or a lightweight medicine ball.

7

BODY-WEIGHT TRAINING

Body-weight exercises are one of the oldest forms of strength training. This type of exercise simply involves using body weight as resistance. Push-ups, pull-ups, and powerful hops, skips, and jumps are examples of body-weight exercises that develop strength and power. Obviously, a major advantage of body-weight training is that you need no equipment, and therefore it is free of cost. Also, children can perform a variety of exercises, and many children can train at the same time. One drawback of body-weight training is the difficulty in adjusting the body weight to the strength level. Some children might not be strong enough to perform even a single push-up, whereas other children might be able to perform 20 repetitions or more.

Like other types of strength training, body-weight training can be a safe and effective method of conditioning, provided that children learn how to perform the exercises correctly. In our programs we want children to experience success while strength training, so we carefully choose the body-weight exercises that are appropriate for each child's strength level. For example, if we are working with a group of overweight children who have never strength trained before, we may use only one or two body-weight exercises for the legs and abdominals and use adjustable weights for upper-body conditioning. Asking an out-of-shape child to attempt one pull-up in front of his or her friends is not only an ineffective method of strength training but also a potentially

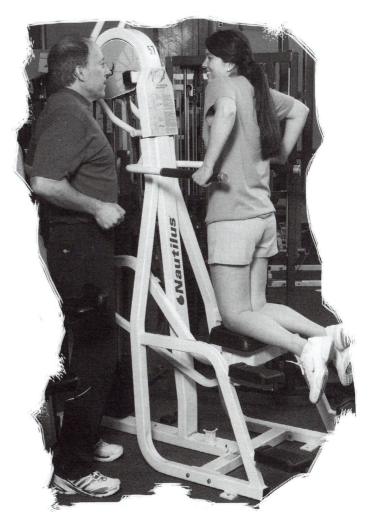

Weight-assisted machines enable youth to perform body weight exercises.

humiliating experience. Conversely, an aspiring young athlete may be able to perform powerful hops and jumps with vigor.

Once children develop enough strength to handle their body weight, it is possible to develop a total-body workout using body-weight exercises. We have found body-weight circuit training to be a safe, effective, and inexpensive method of training for young athletes. In this method of training, children move from one body-weight exercise to the next with about a minute of rest between exercises. However, this type of training can be aerobically taxing; therefore you should gradually increase the intensity of training and carefully monitor the rest interval between exercises. That is, give children an opportunity to learn new exercises and adapt to the demands of the training stimulus before the program becomes too challenging and unpleasant. Over time, you can add exercises and reduce the rest periods between exercises.

Using Body Weight as Resistance

There are two basic types of body-weight training: strength training and power training. Push-ups and curl-ups are examples of more traditional strength-building exercises that are common in most youth strength-training programs. The principles of performing body-weight strength exercises are the same as for other strength-training methods: Children should warm up before they strength train and should always wear appropriate attire (including athletic shoes). Children should perform strength-building exercises in a controlled manner throughout the full range of motion and should breathe continuously during the exercise. Body-weight strength exercises provide children with an opportunity to enhance their muscular strength while developing useful upper-body and lower-body movement skills. In our youth programs, children first learn how to perform body-weight strength exercises at a controlled speed before attempting to perform exercises that require faster speeds and power.

Body-weight power training is recognized as an effective method of conditioning for adults, but current research suggests that this type of training can also provide a distinct advantage for youth. Unlike body-weight strength exercises, power exercises such as jumps and hops are performed explosively. This type of power training, also called plyometric training, conditions the body through dynamic movements that involve a rapid stretch of a muscle (called an eccentric muscle action), which is immediately followed by a rapid shortening of the same muscle (called a concentric muscle action). Although both types of muscle actions are important for the performance of a plyometric exercise, the amount of time it takes to change direction from the eccentric muscle action to the concentric muscle action is a critical factor in power training. Even common playground activities such as hopscotch can be considered a form of plyometric training. When a child jumps from square to square, the quadricep muscles stretch when the child lands and then shorten when the child jumps. Although gamelike in nature, this type of activity actually conditions the body to increase speed of movement and improve power production.

> Plyometric training conditions the body through dynamic movements that involve a rapid stretch of a muscle (called an eccentric muscle action), which is immediately followed by a rapid shortening of the same muscle (called a concentric muscle action).

When properly performed, a plyometric exercise enables a muscle to reach maximal force in the shortest possible time. When the stretching and shortening of a muscle are performed quickly, the force generated during the muscle action is greater than the force that would be generated if the muscle was not stretched immediately before the muscle action. Think about a young basketball player who attempts to block a shot during a game. The athlete bends his knees (stretching phase) and then quickly reverses direction and jumps as high as he can to block the shot (shortening phase). Without the muscle-stretching phase immediately preceding the muscle-shortening phase, he would not jump as high.

Regular plyometric training can actually make youth faster and more powerful by training the neuromuscular system to react more quickly to the stretch-shortening cycle. Indeed, childhood may be the ideal time to incorporate plyometric training into a fitness program because the neuromuscular system of children can readily adapt to this type of training stress. Although adults can benefit from plyometric training, the so-called skill-hungry years for learning motor skills that involve jumping, hopping, skipping, and throwing occur during childhood and early adolescence. As such, a child who does not perform this type of conditioning may have difficulty catching up when the time comes to participate in more advanced training programs.

Well-planned and well-implemented power-training programs can help youth develop movement competence by enhancing their ability to jump, hop, skip, and throw. In our youth programs, the development of athletic qualities through fundamental movement skills serves as the foundation for later success in sports. Perhaps it is not surprising to note that the best athletes learn how to perform complex movement skills early in life. Because training adaptations are specific to the movement pattern, it is easy to see that youth who properly perform plyometric exercises will become more powerful.

Keep in mind that plyometric training needs to be carefully prescribed and consistent with each child's needs and abilities. A major concern we have with many plyometric training programs is that they are too advanced for youth, who are physically and psychologically less mature than adults. For this reason, it is important to gradually progress from simple to more complex exercises and focus on the quality of each movement instead of the quantity. Once movement speed or exercise technique begins to falter, stop the exercise and take a break. Since muscles are required to function at a higher level during plyometric training than for other modes of exercise, specific guidelines for youth plyometric training are outlined in the sidebar.

Body-Weight Exercises

Begin with exercises that are less demanding and progress to exercises that are more challenging as strength and power improve. In some cases, it might be necessary to modify an exercise to make it easier to perform. For example, performing a push-up from the knees or against a wall may be appropriate for some children who find the standard push-up too difficult. Similarly, it makes sense to introduce youth to body-weight power training with less intense double-leg jumps rather than more challenging single-leg hops. These modified versions work the same muscle groups but are less demanding and therefore more

TRAINING GUIDELINES FOR YOUTH PLYOMETRICS

- Begin each session with a 5- to 10-minute dynamic warm-up period.
- Perform plyometric exercises early in the workout when the body is fresh.
- Initially perform 1 or 2 sets of 6 to 8 repetitions on upper- and lower-body exercises.
- Begin with lower-intensity drills and gradually progress to higher-intensity drills.
- Perform each exercise at a fast tempo while focusing on proper exercise technique.
- Allow adequate recovery between sets to maximize muscle performance.
- Systematically vary the training program over time to optimize gains and reduce boredom.
- Perform plyometric training two nonconsecutive days per week.
- Wear supportive athletic footwear.
- Perform lower-body exercises on a surface that has some resilience.
- Regularly provide participants with information on proper training procedures.

consistent with the needs and abilities of school-age youth who may have limited experience performing body-weight exercises.

> It might be necessary to modify an exercise to make it easier to perform. For example, performing a push-up from the knees or against a wall may be appropriate for some children who find the standard push-up too difficult.

You can use body-weight exercises to train all the major muscle groups. After a dynamic warm-up, begin with exercises that children can comfortably perform for the desired number of repetitions and gradually increase the difficulty of the exercise over time. Whenever possible, we introduce new drills based on exercises that the participants already know because children learn more quickly when they are somewhat familiar with the movement patterns being taught. For example, once children learn how to perform a body-weight squat, we might introduce a power exercise such as a squat jump, which requires the lower-body muscles to function at a higher level. Once children gain competence and confidence in their abilities to perform body-weight strength exercises, they should perform power exercises before strength-building exercises. Otherwise, muscles will be fatigued and less capable of generating near-maximal power.

The body-weight exercises are organized into two sections: strength exercises and power (or plyometric) exercises. The specific muscles used are listed for the strength exercises, whereas no muscles are listed for the power exercises because they are total body movements that involve all muscles of the lower body. Upper-body power exercises with medicine balls are described in chapter 6.

BODY-WEIGHT SQUAT

Muscles

Quadriceps, gluteals, hamstrings

Procedure

1. Begin by standing erect with your feet about hip-width apart and toes pointing slightly outward. Place your hands on your hips or straight out in front of your body.

2. Slowly bend your ankles, knees, and hips until your thighs are parallel to the floor. Keep your back flat, head up, and eyes fixed straight ahead. Pause briefly in the bottom position.

3. Return to starting position by slowly straightening your knees and hips.

Technique Tips

- Your knees should follow a slightly outward pattern of the feet. Do not let the knees cave in.

- Avoid bouncing out of the bottom position.

- Concentrate on keeping your head up and chest out. Avoid excessive forward lean.

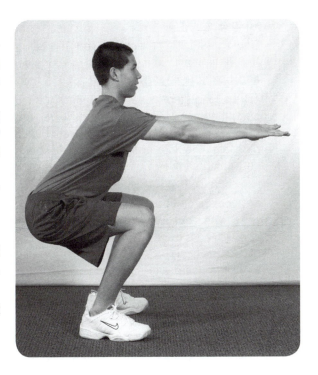

BODY-WEIGHT LUNGE

Muscles

Quadriceps, hamstrings, gluteals

Procedure

1. Begin by standing erect with your feet about hip-width apart. Hold your arms at your sides and look straight forward.

2. Take a long step forward with your right leg; bend the knee of the right leg and lower your body. The thigh of the right leg should be parallel to the floor, and the right knee should be over the ankle of the right foot. Bend the left knee slightly.

3. Lift your body upward slightly, and step forward with your left leg. Bring your left leg forward, and lower your body until the thigh of your left leg is parallel to the floor. Continue to walk forward, alternating legs.

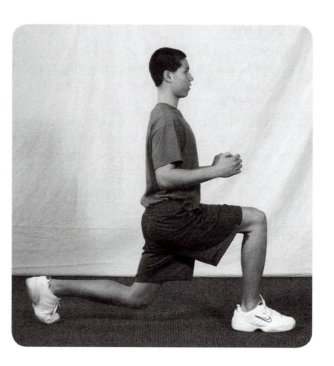

Technique Tips

- Keep your head up, back upright, and shoulders over hips.

- This exercise requires balance and coordination. Take your time to learn the proper form.

- Avoid using upper-torso momentum to return to the starting position. Concentrate on keeping your back upright throughout the exercise.

BODY-WEIGHT HEEL RAISE

Muscles

Gastrocnemius, soleus

Procedure

1. Begin by standing erect with your feet about hip-width apart. Place the ball of the right foot on a board or step with the heel off the surface. Use the free left hand for balance by holding on to the wall or banister. Wrap the left foot around the right ankle.

2. Rise onto the right toe as high as possible with right knee straight; then slowly lower the heel as far as comfortable. Complete the assigned number of repetitions, and repeat with opposite leg.

Technique Tips

• Concentrate on keeping your torso and knees straight to avoid upper-leg involvement.

• If this exercise is too difficult, you can perform it with both feet on a board or step.

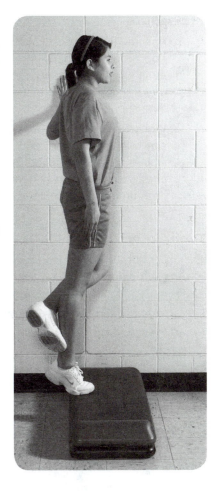

PUSH-UP

Muscles

Pectoralis major, deltoids, triceps

Procedure

1. Assume a prone position on the floor with your body straight, arms fully extended, legs slightly apart, and hands slightly more than shoulder-width apart.

2. While keeping your back flat, slowly lower your body until your elbows are at 90 degrees. Pause briefly, then push away from the floor until you fully extend your arms.

Technique Tips

- Do not allow the hips to sag or rise up during this exercise.

- For variety, place hands in slightly wider or narrower starting position.

Modifications

If this exercise is too difficult, try a wall push-up or a bent-knee push-up. To perform a wall push-up, stand about 2 feet (0.6 m) from a wall and place your hands slightly wider than shoulder-width apart on the wall. Slowly lower your body close to the wall, pause briefly, then return to starting position.

To perform a 90-degree bent-knee push-up, lie facedown on the floor with your body straight and hands slightly wider than shoulder-width apart. Bend your knees to 90 degrees and keep your feet close together. The weight of your body should be on your hands and knees. Support your body with your arms fully extended. Slowly lower your body until your elbows are to 90 degrees. Pause briefly and then push away from the floor until you fully extend your arms.

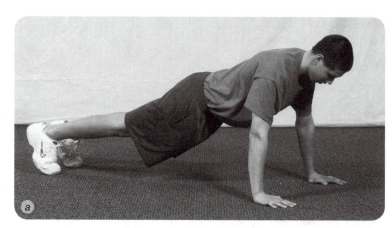

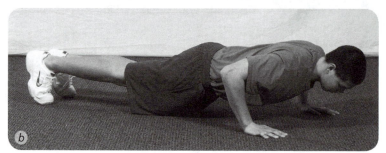

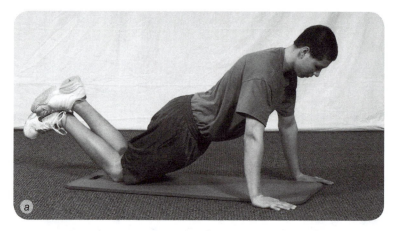

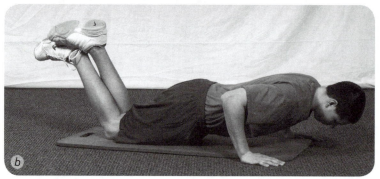

CHIN-UP

Muscles

Latissimus dorsi, biceps

Procedure

1. Grasp a bar overhead with arms extended and torso straight. Hands should be about shoulder-width apart and palms should face your body.
2. Pull your body upward until your chin is above the bar. Lower your body to the starting position.

Technique Tips

- If you need assistance with this exercise, a spotter can help by placing his or her hands on your waist to help lift your body upward.

- Be careful when letting go of the bar. If necessary, an adult spotter should provide assistance.

- For variety, try a wide-grip pull-up with your palms facing away from your body.

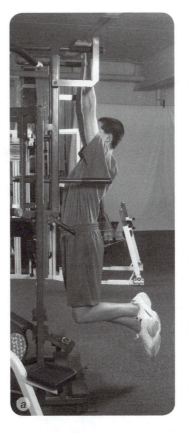
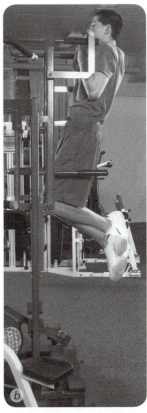

Modifications

- For some children, chin-ups and pull-ups may be too difficult. In this case, begin with a front pull-down on a weight machine or a chin-up on a weight-assisted chin-dip machine that reduces body weight by a counterweight system.

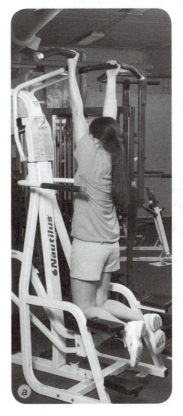
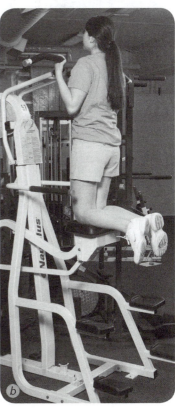

BAR DIP

Muscles

Triceps, pectoralis major, deltoids

Procedure

1. Grip the dip bar with palms facing each other and arms fully extended. Keep your body straight.

2. Slowly lower your body until the elbows are at right angles. Then push upward to the starting position.

Technique Tips

- Avoid swinging your body during this exercise, and do not bounce out of the bottom position.

- Do not flex the elbows beyond 90 degrees.

- If your feet touch the floor, cross your lower legs.

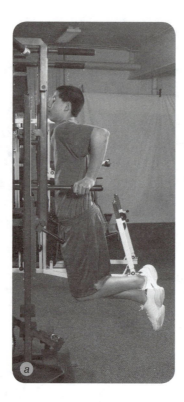

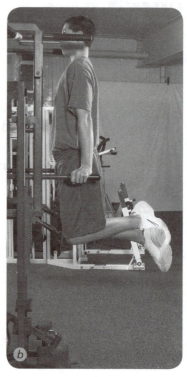

Modifications

If you cannot complete a dip with the proper technique, use a weight-assisted chin-dip machine with an adjustable weight stack (*a-b*) or a chair dip (*c*). To perform a chair dip, while facing away from a chair place the heels of your hand about shoulder-width apart on the front edge of a chair or bench. Fully extend your elbows so your arms are straight. Your fingers should point backward, and your legs should be straight with both feet on the floor. Slowly lower your body until your elbows form right angles. Then return to the starting position. Make sure the chair or bench is secure so that it will not slip during this exercise.

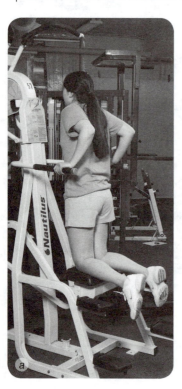

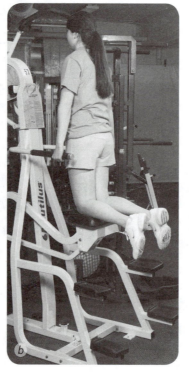

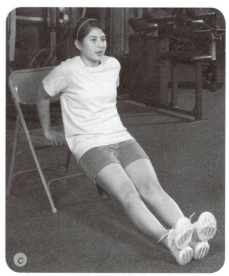

TRUNK CURL AND DIAGONAL TRUNK CURL

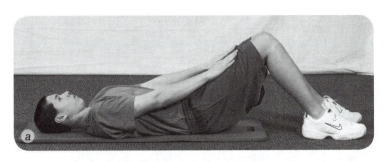

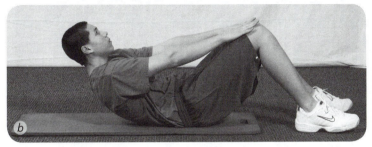

Muscles

Rectus abdominis, internal oblique, external oblique

Procedure

1. Lie on the floor with your knees bent and feet on the floor. Place your hands on your thighs with your arms fully extended.

2. Slowly curl your shoulders and upper back off the floor while sliding your hands up your thighs. Keep your lower back on the floor. Your hands should reach your kneecaps.

3. Pause momentarily, then return to the starting position.

4. To perform a diagonal curl, which emphasizes the obliques on the sides of the midsection, reach your left hand toward your right kneecap, and slowly return to starting position; then reach your right hand toward your left kneecap.

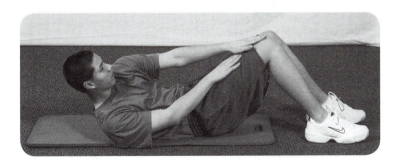

Technique Tips

- You can place both hands across your chest or behind your head during this exercise. If you place your hands behind your head, be careful not to pull your head forward with your hands during the exercise.

- Your lower back should remain in contact with the floor during these exercises.

HANGING KNEE RAISE

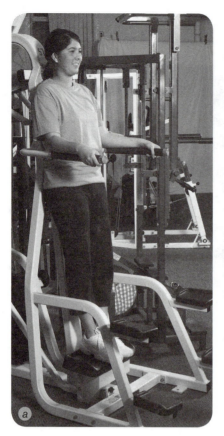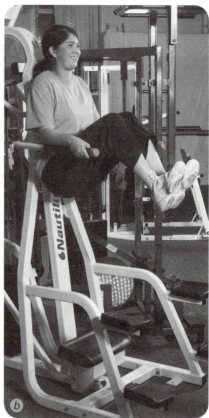

Muscles
Rectus abdominis, hip flexor

Procedure
1. Grasp the dip bars with both hands, place your forearms on the pads, and let your body hang. Place your back against the support.
2. Begin the movement by lifting your bent knees toward your chest. Pause briefly and then lower the legs to the starting position.

Technique Tips
- Keep your back and arms motionless during this exercise.
- Exhale as you lift your knees towards your chest.

PELVIC TILT

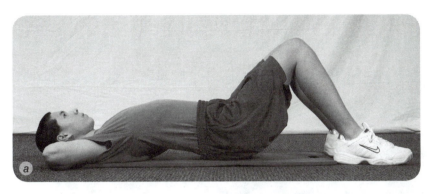

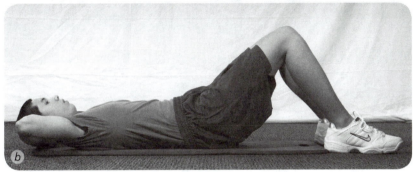

Muscle
Rectus abdominis

Procedure
1. Lie on the floor with your knees bent and feet on the floor. Place your hands loosely behind your head.
2. Slowly press your lower back against the floor by tightening your abdominals. Hold this position for 5 seconds; return to the starting position.

Technique Tip
Breathe normally throughout this exercise.

KNEELING HIP EXTENSION

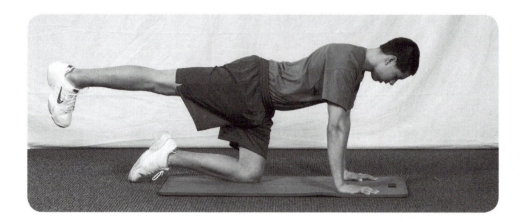

Muscles

Erector spinae, hip extensors

Procedure

1. Kneel on the floor, supporting your body on both hands and both knees.
2. Slowly extend your right leg backward until it is parallel to the floor. Pause momentarily, then return your right leg to the starting position and extend your left leg backward. Pause momentarily, then return your left leg to the starting position and continue to alternate legs.

Technique Tips

- Perform this exercise in a slow and controlled manner. Do not raise your limbs higher than parallel to the floor and keep your shoulders and hips level.
- For a more challenging exercise known as the quadruped, raise your left arm parallel to the floor while you extend your right leg (and vice versa).

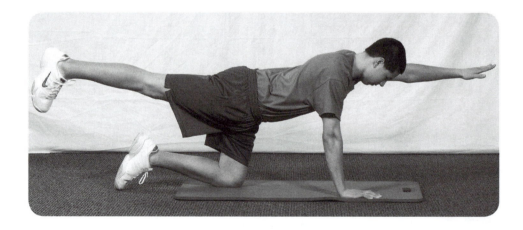

PRONE PLANK

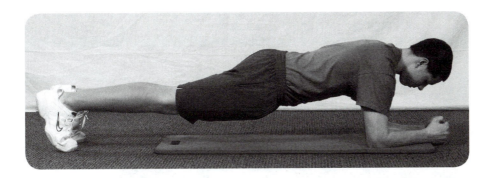

Muscles

Rectus abdominis, internal oblique, external oblique

Procedure

1. Lie facedown on the floor with legs extended, supporting your body on both forearms.
2. Keep back flat and head in line with torso. Hold position for the desired duration (e.g., 10 to 30 seconds).

Technique Tips

- Breathe normally as you hold the position.
- Activate the abdominal muscles to maintain the correct body position.

SIDE PLANK

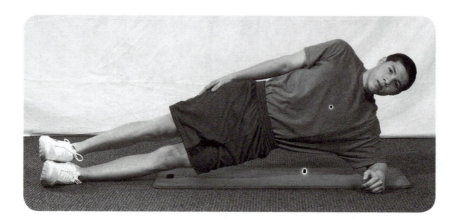

Muscles

Rectus abdominis, internal oblique, external oblique

Procedure

1. Lie on your left side with your left elbow under your left shoulder and support your body with your left forearm (and vice versa).

2. Keep your body straight and head in line with your torso. Hold position for the desired duration (e.g., 10 to 30 seconds).

Technique Tips

- Breathe normally as you hold the position.
- Activate the abdominal muscles to maintain the correct body position.

ANKLE JUMP

Procedure

1. Stand with feet about shoulder-width apart.
2. Using only the ankles to generate momentum, jump up and down in one place.
3. Land with knees slightly bent and repeat.

Technique Tips

- Extend both ankles to the maximum range of motion on every jump.
- Try to get as high as possible with every jump.

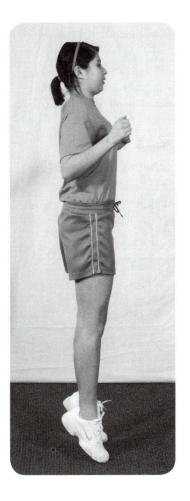

JUMP AND FREEZE

Procedure

1. Stand with feet about shoulder-width apart.

2. Bend at the knees and quickly jump as far forward as possible. Hold landing position for 2 to 3 seconds and then repeat.

Technique Tips

- Use both arms to assist in the forward jumping movement.

- Land with both feet on the ground and knees slightly bent.

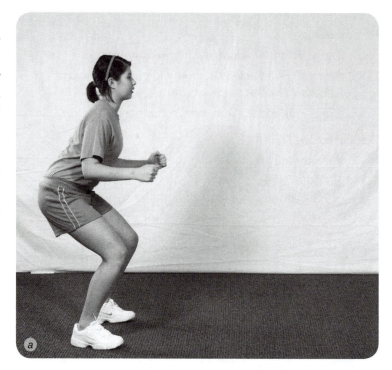

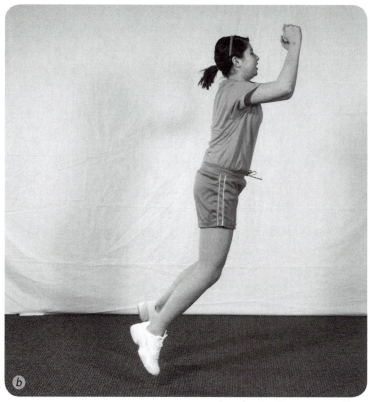

BACKWARD JUMP AND FREEZE

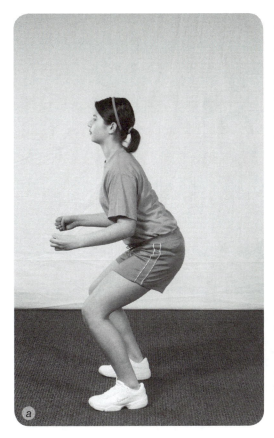
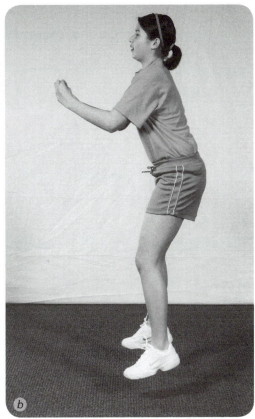

Procedure

1. Stand with feet about shoulder-width apart.
2. Bend at the knees and jump backward, keeping the elbows at 90 degrees for body control. Hold landing position for 2 to 3 seconds and then repeat.

Technique Tips

- Keep your chest over toes to avoid falling backward.
- Focus on the control of the jump rather than the distance of the jump.

STANDING JUMP AND REACH

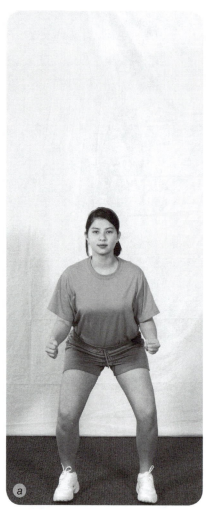
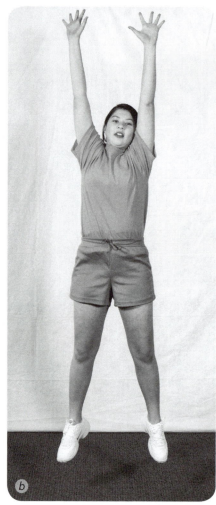

Procedure

1. Stand with feet about shoulder-width apart.
2. Bend at the knees and quickly jump upward, reaching as high as possible.
3. Land with knees bent and repeat.

Technique Tips

- Use both arms to assist in the upward jumping movement.
- Land softly with knees bent and both feet on the ground.
- For variety, perform this jump next to a partner and give each other a high five at the top of every jump.

CONE JUMP

Procedure

1. Set up a series of cones in a row spaced about 18 to 24 inches (46 to 61 cm) apart.

2. Rapidly jump forward over each cone, keeping your body vertical.

3. Land with knees slightly bent and repeat.

Technique Tips

- Use both arms to maintain balance and assist in the upward jumping movement.

- Try to spend as little time on the ground as possible.

- Use additional cones or taller cones to make this exercise more challenging.

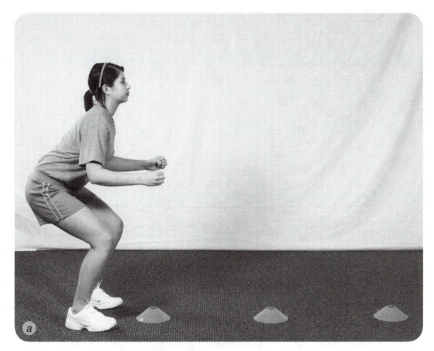

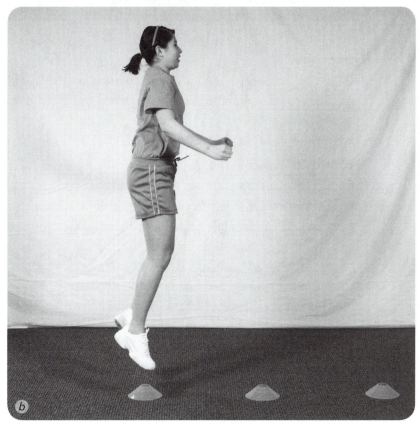

LATERAL CONE JUMP

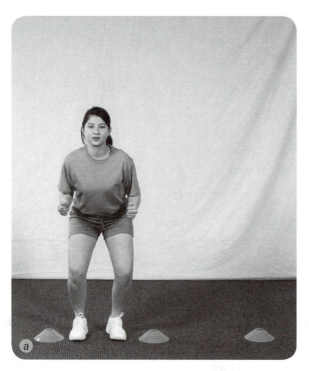
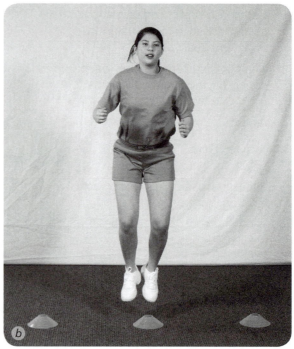

Procedure

1. Set up a series of cones in a row spaced about 18 to 24 inches (46 to 61 cm) apart.
2. Stand perpendicular to the cones and then rapidly jump sideways over each cone, keeping your body vertical.
3. Land with knees slightly bent and repeat.

Technique Tips

- Use both arms to maintain balance and assist in the jumping movement.
- Try to spend as little time on the ground as possible.
- Use additional cones or taller cones to make this exercise more challenging.

ZIGZAG JUMP

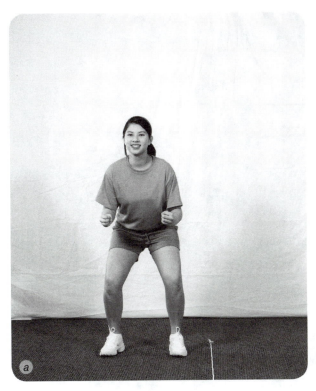

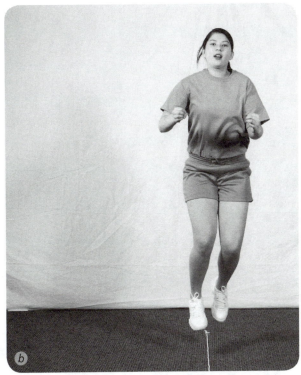

Procedure

1. Use a line on the playing field or set up a long rope on the floor.
2. Stand at one end of the line with both feet on the same side.
3. Jump and land on the other side of the line while moving forward; then immediately jump to the other side and repeat.

Technique Tips

- Use both arms to maintain balance and assist in the jumping movement.
- Land with both knees slightly bent.
- Jump as far down the line as possible.
- Hop on one leg back and forth to make this exercise more challenging.

90-DEGREE JUMP

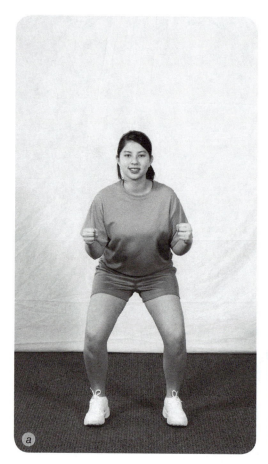 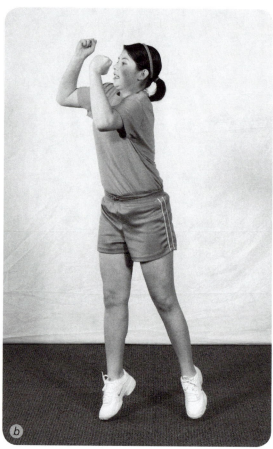

Procedure

1. Stand with your feet about shoulder-width apart while facing an object as a point of reference.

2. Jump as high as you can; while in the air, turn 90 degree to the right. Land and immediately repeat the jump, turning 90 degrees back to the left.

Technique Tips

- Use both arms to maintain balance and assist in the jumping movement.
- Land with both knees slightly bent.

SQUARE JUMP

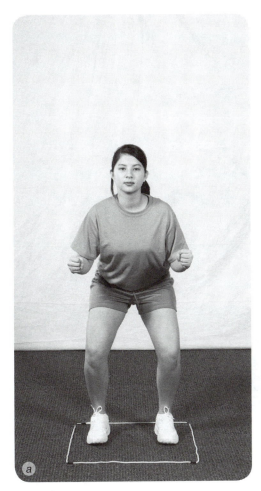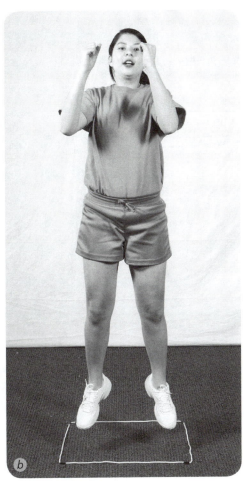

Procedure

1. Set up four strips of tape or rope, each 24 inches (61 cm) long, in the shape of a square on the floor.
2. Stand in the center of the square with your feet shoulder-width apart.
3. Jump forward over the line straight in front of you, then immediately jump back to the starting position. While looking forward, jump sideways and backward over each line, returning to the middle of the square after each jump.

Technique Tips

- Use both arms to maintain balance and assist in the jumping movement.
- Land with both knees slightly bent.
- For variety, change the order of the jumps.

POWER SKIPPING

Procedure

1. Stand with feet shoulder-width apart and both arms at 90 degrees.
2. Skip forward, lifting opposite knee and arm to maximize height.

Technique Tips

- Spend as little time on the ground as possible, trying to maximize hang time by emphasizing upward knee drive.
- Focus on full ankle extension with each skip.

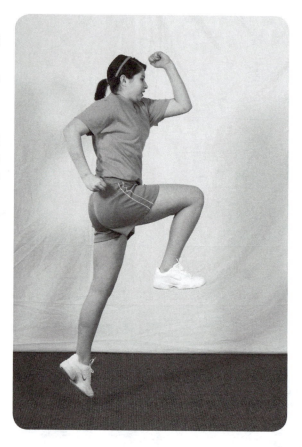

Summary

Although body-weight training does not require expensive equipment, this type of training requires competent instruction and a careful choice of exercises because some children might not have enough strength to perform body-weight exercises correctly. Therefore, we take the time to choose body-weight exercises that are appropriate for each child's fitness level to ensure successful performance and positive reinforcement. It is essential for children to experience success and feel good about their performance. If necessary, modify a traditional exercise in order to make it easier to perform. Give children an opportunity to learn about body-weight training and gradually add new strength and power exercises to their exercise program. Although it may take a little longer to master proper technique on a body-weight exercise than on a single-joint weight machine exercise, this type of training requires greater balance, coordination, and stabilization, which make body-weight training so beneficial for children and teenagers. Many body-weight exercises can be used in enhancing the strength and power of beginners as well as young athletes.

PART III

PROGRAM DESIGN

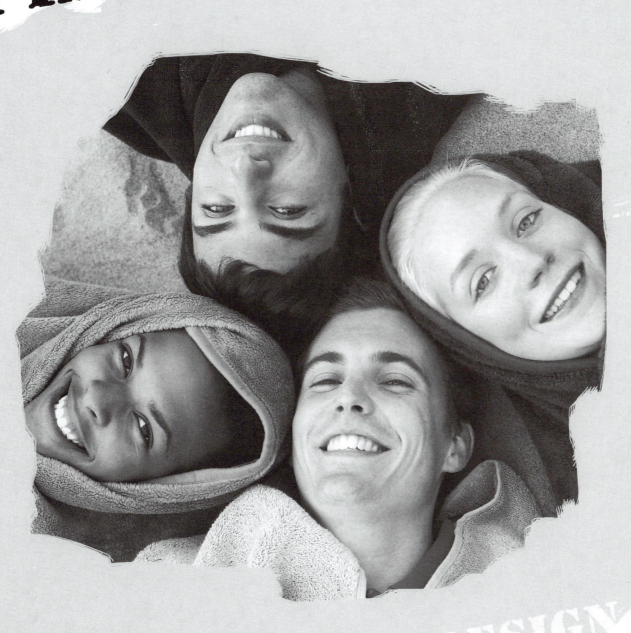

GENERAL PREPARATION

8

In the past, the focus of most physical education classes and youth activity programs was on the development of sport-specific skills. But now it appears that involvement in a variety of health-enhancing physical activities is necessary for maximizing physical fitness and enhancing sport performance. Specializing in one sport or skill at a young age not only places late-maturing youth at a disadvantage, but it also increases the risk of sport-related injuries, which are a significant cause of hospitalization and health care costs during childhood and adolescence. This is why it is so important to enhance muscular fitness during physical education classes and sport practice. When youngsters have well-conditioned muscles, they will be better prepared for all types of physical activity and more successful in mastering the motor skills required for higher levels of sport performance. Furthermore, they are more likely to enjoy physical activity, and their risk of suffering a sport-related injury is reduced. With these things in mind, it should be obvious that strength training is a fundamental fitness activity for all boys and girls.

Preparatory Conditioning

Children need to participate regularly in some supervised strength-building activities as part of a well-rounded physical activity program. Although the concept of strength training for youth may seem unnecessary to some parents and teachers, in a growing number of cases the musculoskeletal system of boys and girls is poorly prepared for the demands of recreational physical activity and sport practice. Participation in preparatory strength and conditioning activities is particularly important for sedentary youth and should be a standard procedure for aspiring young athletes in preparing them for more successful performance and reducing their risk of suffering sport-related injuries. Despite the focus on early specialization in specific sports in some communities, participation in physical activity should not begin with sport practice and competition but should evolve out of preparatory conditioning and instructional practice sessions that are gradually progressed over time.

> Participation in preparatory strength and conditioning activities is particularly important for sedentary youth and should be a standard procedure for aspiring young athletes in preparing them for more successful performance and reducing their risk of suffering sport-related injuries.

Although some young athletes believe that they can play themselves into shape, the specific benefits of strength training cannot be realized without actual participation in a strength-training program. We now have a better understanding of the effects of strength exercise in youth, and we realize that regular participation in a strength-training program that is individually prescribed and systematically varied over time can play an important role in optimizing athletic performance and reducing the risk of sport-related injuries. According to some sports medicine professionals, up to 50 percent of overuse injuries in youth sports could be prevented if young athletes strengthened their muscles, bones, and connective tissue before focusing on sport-specific training. Soccer fields and basketball courts are filled with children whose musculoskeletal systems are not prepared for two hours of sport training five or more days per week. While all young athletes will likely benefit from strength exercise, preparatory conditioning that includes strength training has proven to be particularly beneficial for young female athletes who appear to be more susceptible to knee injuries than young male athletes.

Children who are already active in organized sports may need to make some training adjustments before adding strength exercise to an already full schedule of physical pursuits. To prevent overtraining and permit appropriate recovery time, carefully evaluate the young athlete's weekly training program. For example, a young basketball player should incorporate strength training into a redesigned workout schedule rather than simply add it to the weekly training routine. While the potential benefits of preparatory conditioning are remarkable, a downfall of some youth programs is insufficient recovery time between training sessions. A reduction in performance and an increased risk of injury will likely be the consequence of frequent training sessions with inadequate recovery between workouts.

Teachers and coaches who work with youth need to pay special attention to the intensity and volume of the exercise program as well as the amount of rest and recovery between exercise sessions if injury reduction is a primary training objective. In short, strength training should not simply be added into a youngster's training program but rather sensibly incorporated into a multifactorial conditioning program that varies throughout the year. In a growing number of cases, aspiring young athletes may need to reduce the amount of time they spend practicing sport-specific skills to allow time for participation in strength and conditioning activities. It is noteworthy that most researchers and clinicians who observed significant benefits of preparatory strength and conditioning employed a training frequency of two or three nonconsecutive days per week.

Training Youth

Physical measures of strength and power will improve throughout childhood and adolescence simply as the result of growth and maturation. For example, push-up scores and vertical jump performance will increase over time as the result of biological development even without participation in a structured strength-training program. As such, children cannot be treated

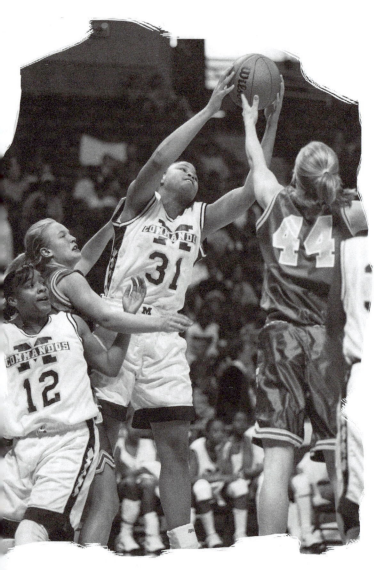

Strength training can reduce the risk of injury in young athletes, thus giving them more playing time.

as miniature adults, because their physiology is dynamic. Even though regular participation in a strength-training program will enhance the strength and power of youth above and beyond growth and development, coaches and teachers need to understand that children and adolescents are in a constant state of change. Thus, training programs that are appropriate for adult athletes would likely be too demanding for youth who are still growing and developing.

Figure 8.1 illustrates the possible outcomes of strength training in children and adolescents. Curve A represents normal improvements in muscle strength as the result of growth and development, whereas curve B illustrates training-induced gains that are possible through regular participation in a strength-training program. As illustrated on curve B, a child who participates in a progressive strength-training program will have better strength performance at any age when compared to an age-matched peer who does not strength train. Furthermore, it is reasonable to assume that strength training throughout childhood and adolescence will build a foundation for even greater gains in strength and power during adulthood. Conversely, arduous training sessions with inadequate recovery between workouts and sport practice might result in frustration, burnout, or even injury. Curve C is an example of what might happen when the demands of strength training and sport practice exceed the physical abilities of youth. An understanding of the possible outcomes of strength training on youth will assist in the design of fitness programs that enhance the ultimate strength performance of young weight trainers.

Although a day off between workouts may be adequate for beginners who participate in single-set training programs with a light to moderate load, strength training to enhance sport performance involves higher levels of physical as well as psychological stress. Therefore, well-planned activities are required for maximizing recovery and returning to an optimal performance state. This is particularly important for young athletes who represent different sport teams or participate in extracurricular conditioning activities at private training centers. In some cases, youth coaches may not be aware of the cumulative stress placed on children in their sport programs. When people of any age participate in a strength-training program, it is important to understand and genuinely appreciate the relationship between exercise and recovery in order to optimize training adaptations. Additional information on program variation and long-term planning is discussed in chapter 13.

> Although a day off between workouts may be adequate for beginners who participate in single-set training programs with a light to moderate load, strength training to enhance sport performance involves higher levels of physical as well as psychological stress. Therefore, well-planned activities are required for maximizing recovery and returning to an optimal performance state.

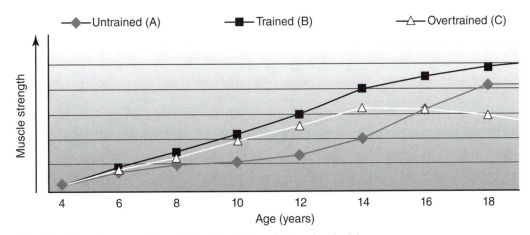

Figure 8.1 Possible outcomes of strength training during childhood and adolescence.

Adapted from T. Rowland, 2005, *Children's exercise physiology*, 2nd ed. (Champaign, IL: Human Kinetics), XII.

Dynamic Motivation

Getting youth ready for strength training is not just about static stretching. A well-designed dynamic warm-up can set the tone for the training session and establish the desired tempo for the upcoming activities. If a warm-up is slow and monotonous, then performance during the main physical activities that follow may be less than expected. However, if the warm-up is up-tempo, varied, and exciting, performance during the strength-training session will likely meet or exceed expectations. In addition, warm-up activities that are active, engaging, and challenging and provide an opportunity for children to gain confidence in their abilities to perform fundamental movement skills are far more enjoyable than traditional stretch-and-hold activities, which many children find boring. In short, the warm-up period should satisfy the need for students to move when they enter the gymnasium as well as to focus their attention on listening and learning.

> A well-designed dynamic warm-up can set the tone for the training session and establish the desired tempo for the upcoming activities.

Although warm-up protocols that include static stretching have become standard practice, over the past few years long-held beliefs about the potential benefits of warm-up static stretching have been questioned. There has been a growing interest in warm-up procedures that involve the performance of dynamic hops, skips, jumps, and lunges designed to elevate body temperature, enhance the excitability of muscle fibers, improve kinesthetic awareness, and maximize active ranges of motion. During a dynamic exercise, the muscles are stretched to a new range of motion and then forced to contract to perform the desired action. Since muscles are actually used in a new range of motion, it is logical to assume that they will be better prepared for strength-training activities. It is important to understand that a dynamic stretch does not involve a bouncing-type movement that is characteristic of a ballistic stretch but rather a controlled elongation of specific muscle groups.

We begin physical education classes and youth fitness programs with a 10-minute warm-up period that typically consists of 8 to 10 drills that progress from relatively simple movements to more challenging exercises that involve more complex movement patterns. Children and teens perform each dynamic movement for about 10 yards (9 m), rest about 5 to 10 seconds, and then repeat the same exercise for 10 yards as they return to the starting point. Alternatively, students can move around the gymnasium as they perform different dynamic activities. Our goal is to integrate a variety of movements into our dynamic warm-up protocols rather than isolate specific stretches or muscles. Following our demonstration, children perform each exercise as we provide instruction on maintaining proper form (e.g., vertical torso, knees toward chest, up on toes). In our physical education classes and afterschool fitness programs, there is a seamless transition from our dynamic warm-up to the start of the main strength-training workout.

Since youth see little value in prolonged periods of aerobic exercise, a dynamic warm-up is more consistent with how children naturally move: short bursts of moderate- to high-intensity physical activity interspersed with brief periods of rest as needed. Since equipment is not necessary, dynamic warm-up protocols are a cost-effective method for enhancing the fundamental movement skills of games and sports. Furthermore, data from our youth fitness center indicate that the heart rate response to dynamic exercise averages about 150 beats per minute. As such, dynamic warm-up protocols may increase the amount of time children engage in moderate to vigorous physical activity, which is an important public health objective.

During our warm-up sessions, we want participants to do more than increase body temperature. We want to prime their neuromuscular systems for the main activity portion of the physical education or sport lesson. We refer to this sequence as warm up, turn on, and work out. *Warm up* refers to exercises and drills that prepare the children for the lesson. Instead of static stretching, we use a variety of dynamic activities that require balance, agility, coordination, flexibility, strength, and power. *Turn on* refers to activation of the neuromuscular system to excite the proper musculature. Since most kids have been sitting in school before physical education or sport practice, their muscles need to be turned on for the main activity component of the lesson. This is accomplished by the performance of low-, moderate-, and high-intensity dynamic movements. *Work out* refers to the conditioning aspect of our warm-up protocols that can result in meaningful improvements in functional stability, fundamental movement skills, and fitness performance. Thus, a well-designed dynamic warm-up can enhance physical fitness and prepare the body for more vigorous movements that occur during some physical education lessons and sport practice workouts.

A principle of our dynamic warm-up protocol is that the exercises are similar in design and function to the activities the kids will perform in the main activity segment of physical education classes and fitness workouts. While we recognize the value of traditional stretch-and-hold exercises, we incorporate static stretching exercises into the cool-down rather than the warm-up period. Remember that the goal of traditional stretching is to relax the muscles, whereas the goal of a dynamic warm-up is to activate the muscles. During the performance of a dynamic exercise, not only do muscles lengthen (as they do in a static stretch), but they also contract and move in an enhanced range of motion.

A dynamic warm-up routine we use for school-age youth is outlined in table 8.1 on page 174. Since there are literally hundreds of exercises that can be incorporated into a dynamic warm-up, the sample exercises should be used as a starting point or a guide to help you develop a routine that is consistent with the needs and abilities of children and adolescents you work with. Although a dynamic warm-up may feel like a workout, remember that the goal of a dynamic warm-up is to prepare children for the main activity segment of a session without undue fatigue.

As mentioned earlier, we incorporate static stretching exercises into the cool-down rather than the warm-up. Postexercise stretching can facilitate improvements in range of motion because of the increase in muscle temperature. During the cool-down, participants should perform several static stretching exercises for their upper and lower bodies. In addition, during this period it is often worthwhile for participants to reflect on what they learned and for instructors to review training objectives for the next lesson.

Participants should perform each stretch two or three times and hold for about 15 seconds. It is important to remind children to breathe normally while stretching and to reach a point where they feel a gentle pull, not pain. While lots of stretches can be performed during the cool-down session, eight static stretches we use in our youth programs are outlined in table 8.2 on page 175.

Summary

The design of a youth strength-training program involves more than simply prescribing sets and repetitions. Program design involves proper instruction and supervision along with sensible progression, a proper dynamic warm-up, and an understanding that youth are not simply miniature adults. Since physical measures will improve during childhood and adolescence as the result of biological development, a key factor in the design of any youth strength-training program is balancing the demands of training with the need for recovery between workouts. With an age-appropriate prescription of all program variables, strength training can be a worthwhile and enjoyable activity for youth with varied needs, goals, and abilities.

Table 8.1 Sample Dynamic Warm-Up Routine

1. High-knee march		While marching forward or in place, lift left knee toward right elbow, then return to starting position and repeat on opposite side.
2. Stepping trunk turns		With hands clasped behind head, march in place and turn hips to the right 90 degrees then to the left 90 degrees while upper body remains forward.
3. Standing flutter	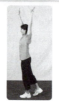	Stand with both arms extended above head and feet shoulder-width apart. Extend left arm and right leg backward a few inches while maintaining an erect body position. Return to starting position and perform with opposite limbs.
4. Low jacks and high jacks		While moving feet apart and together, lift arms from hip to shoulder level. Progress to high jacks by lifting arms from shoulder level to overhead.
5. Inchworm	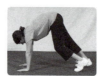	From a push-up position, walk both feet toward the hands with tiny steps while keeping the hips elevated and legs extended. Then return to the starting position by walking the hands forward while keeping arms and legs extended.
6. Giant steps		From a standing position, take a long step forward with your right leg, then step forward with the left leg as far forward as possible.
7. Lateral shuffle		From a standing side stance, lower body to semisquat position, then move laterally by taking a lead step followed by a short secondary step.
8. High-knee skip		Rapidly skip forward while focusing on knee lift, arm action, and reduced ground time.
9. Heel-up		Rapidly move forward while kicking heels toward buttocks.
10. Sprint series		From a standing position, lean forward as you begin to run to the 5-yard mark and then sprint through the 10-yard mark focusing on arm action, knee height, and quick acceleration.

Table 8.2 Static Stretching Exercises

1. Chest stretch		Interlock fingers behind head and gently move elbows backward.
2. Triceps and lat stretch		Reach one arm behind head as if you were trying to scratch your back. Gently pull the elbow toward the midline of your body. Repeat on the other side.
3. Upper-back stretch		Reach across the body with one arm and place the hand on the opposite shoulder. Gently press the elbow across your body. Repeat on the other side.
4. Hamstring stretch	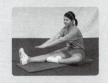	Sit upright on the floor with one leg straight in front of your body and the other knee bent with the heel against the inner thigh of extended leg. Bend at the hip and gently lean forward while keeping extended leg straight. Repeat on the other side.
5. Lower-back and hip stretch		Sit upright on the floor with both legs straight in front of your body. Cross one leg over the other and place opposite arm against the bent knee to assist with torso rotation. Repeat on the other side.
6. Inner-thigh stretch		Sit upright with your knees bent and the soles of your feet touching. Grasp ankles and gently press elbows against knees.
7. Quadriceps stretch	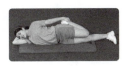	Lie on your side and bend one knee toward buttocks. Grasp the ankle with one hand and gently pull heel toward buttocks. Repeat on the other side.
8. Calf stretch		With arms extended in front of your body, place both hands against a wall for support. Bend the knee of the front leg and keep the back leg straight with the heel on the floor. Repeat on the other side.

9

BASIC STRENGTH AND POWER FOR AGES 7 TO 10

Our research has shown that boys and girls 7 to 10 years of age respond positively and enthusiastically to properly designed strength-training programs. Physiologically, our youngest participants have demonstrated significant gains in their muscle strength and exercise performance. Psychologically, they feel physically competent and self-confident. Above all, children in our strength-training programs have enjoyed exercising in our classes and have acquired skills and knowledge that will result in a lifetime of physical activity.

Despite outdated concerns that strength training was inappropriate or unsafe for children, we are pleased to report that over the past 20 years, there have been no injuries or setbacks among our 7- to 10-year-old trainees. Perhaps just as important, the participants in this age group have had an almost zero dropout rate. When the exercise program is interesting and challenging and the teachers are engaging and motivating, the children seldom miss a session. Typically, the children's attendance rate is over 95 percent, indicating a high level of personal reinforcement from their strength-training efforts.

Instead of prolonged periods of aerobic activities that most children find boring, strength training characterized by short bouts of physical activity interspersed with brief periods of rest can be engaging, challenging, and fun. Furthermore,

if the program starts with simple exercises and gradually progresses to more complex activities, children will begin to value the process of fitness training and regular physical activity. Clearly, childhood is the ideal time to expose boys and girls to a variety of activities they enjoy doing. Fitness testing is important for assessing performance and monitoring progress, but at this age sparking an interest in strength training and physical fitness is just as important.

When introducing children to strength-building activities, instructors and coaches need to explain concepts at a cognitive level they understand. Children should learn that strength training can make muscles and bones stronger and should begin to understand the concept of a fitness workout that includes a warm-up, an exercise session, and a cool-down. Moreover, instructors and coaches need to appreciate each child's training age because what is appropriate for one child might be ineffective or even unsafe for another. For example, an 8-year-old girl who has participated in a strength-training program for one year will likely be able to perform more advanced exercises and lift heavier loads than a 10-year-old girl who has never participated in strength-training activities. In some cases, a child who strength trains regularly may be able to participate in fitness programs designed for teenagers, provided that appropriate training loads are used and qualified coaching is available. Conversely, teenagers who have no experience with strength training may need to begin with simple exercises that are more consistent with their current needs and abilities.

Components of the Warm-Up and Cool-Down

Be sure to begin the strength-training workout with dynamic warm-up activities that feature relays, rope skipping, active games, agility drills, and calisthenics. Use hoops, cones, medicine balls, balloons, and other apparatus to make the warm-up more challenging and to enhance children's movement skills. Not only do dynamic movement exercises during the warm-up period prepare children for strength training exercises, but they also provide an opportunity for boys and girls of all abilities to improve fundamental physical skills such as agility, balance, and coordination.

At the end of a session, cool down with less intense activities and static stretching. At this age, children should be taught a variety of static stretching exercises and should learn how to perform a slow and sustained stretch of the muscles in order to develop and maintain normal range of motion. Since a child with a limited range of motion might have difficulty performing some free-weight and body-weight exercises, it is important to incorporate flexibility activities into the fitness workout.

> Not only do dynamic movement exercises during the warm-up period prepare children for strength training exercises, but they also provide an opportunity for boys and girls of all abilities to improve fundamental physical skills such as agility, balance, and coordination.

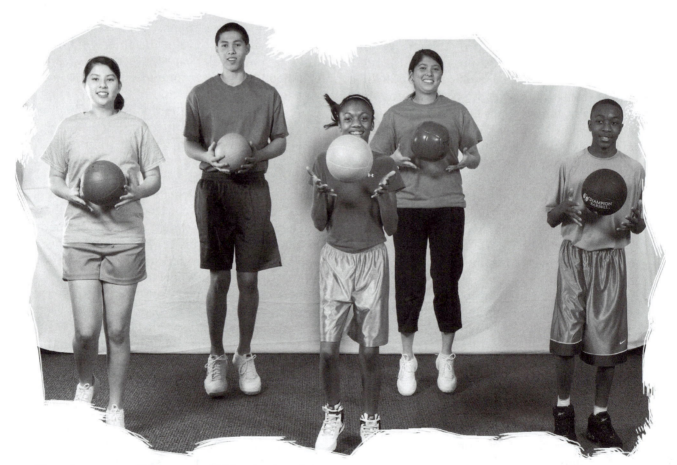

Dynamic warm-up activities prepare children for strength training exercises and improve fundamental physical skills.

Strength-Training Program

The youth strength-training guidelines established by the National Strength and Conditioning Association recommend one to three sets of 6 to 15 repetitions, each with appropriate weight loads. Obviously, weight loads that a person can perform for only 6 repetitions are much heavier than weight loads for 15 repetitions. Likewise, completing three sets of each exercise is more demanding than doing one set of each exercise. Although it is logical to assume that harder workouts produce better results, 7- to 10-year-old boys and girls respond favorably to brief training sessions and make excellent gains in strength by doing more repetitions (about 10 to 15) with moderate weight loads during the first few weeks of strength training.

To condition most major muscle groups, train with 8 to 10 exercises two or three days per week. Some of these, such as the leg press and chest press, work several muscles simultaneously, and others, like the biceps curl and triceps extension, target specific muscles. Children in this age group should use a combination of multiple-muscle and single-muscle exercises that provide comprehensive muscular development. Make sure that children perform every exercise properly and attempt to perform each repetition through a full range of motion.

> Although it is logical to assume that harder workouts produce better results, 7- to 10-year-old boys and girls respond favorably to brief training sessions and make excellent gains in strength by doing more repetitions (about 10 to 15) with moderate weight loads during the first few weeks of strength training.

Instructors and coaches are ultimately responsible for modifying each strength-training workout to match the needs, abilities, and interests of all the children. If the program is boring or too challenging, children will likely develop negative attitudes toward strength training. But with qualified instruction, enthusiastic supervision, and age-appropriate activities, children can learn the basic skills they need for successful and enjoyable participation in a variety of strength-training activities. When teaching children who have never participated in a strength-training program, remember that success is not only measured by assessing gains in muscular fitness but by watching children develop proper exercise technique, progress gradually in difficulty levels, and understand the concept of a fitness workout.

Strength-Training Exercises

Table 9.1 presents sample exercises for 7- to 10-year-olds using child-sized weight-plate machines along with a suggested training protocol. If child-sized weight machines are not available, children can perform a variety of strength exercises safely using free-weight equipment, medicine balls, elastic bands, or body weight. We typically use dumbbells and medicine balls with this age group because they are easy to hold and handle. Thus, children are able to perform exercises such as a dumbbell curl and medicine ball chest pass with more control and confidence. Table 9.2 presents sample strength exercises and training recommendations for 7- to 10-year-olds using dumbbells, and table 9.3 presents sample strength exercises and training recommendations for 7- to 10-year-olds using medicine balls.

While advanced free-weight exercises do not need to be incorporated into all youth resistance-training programs, boys and girls who want to learn weightlifting movements and modified cleans, pulls, and presses might benefit from this type of training if the focus remains on learning proper exercise technique with appropriate loads. Unlike other resistance exercises, lifts such as the power clean and snatch require a high degree of coordination and technical skill. Thus, coaches and teachers must be aware of the considerable amount of time required for teaching these lifts correctly and must be knowledgeable of age-appropriate progression strategies from basic exercises, to skill transfer exercises, and finally to the competitive lifts. Because of the complex nature of these lifts, participants should perform only 3 to 6 repetitions per set of each weightlifting movement. In our youth programs, we begin by developing proper exercise technique with the use of a wooden dowel. Once participants gain

Table 9.1 Child-Sized Machine Exercises for Ages 7 to 10

Exercise	Muscle groups	Sets	Reps
Leg press	Quadriceps Hamstrings Gluteals	1-2	10-15
Leg extension	Quadriceps	1-2	10-15
Leg curl	Hamstrings	1-2	10-15
Chest press	Pectoralis major Front deltoid Triceps	1-2	10-15
Seated row	Latissimus dorsi Rear deltoid Biceps	1-2	10-15
Prone back raise	Erector spinae	1-2	10-15
Trunk curl	Rectus abdominis	1-2	10-15

If desired, progress to 2 sets on selected exercises.

Table 9.2 Dumbbell Exercises for Ages 7 to 10

Exercise	Muscle groups	Sets	Reps
Dumbbell squat	Quadriceps Hamstrings Gluteals	1-2	10-15
Dumbbell lunge	Quadriceps Hamstrings Gluteals	1-2	10-15
Dumbbell step-up	Quadriceps Hamstrings Gluteals	1-2	10-15
Dumbbell bench press	Pectoralis major Front deltoid Triceps	1-2	10-15
Dumbbell one-arm row	Latissimus dorsi Rear deltoid Biceps	1-2	10-15
Dumbbell lateral raise	Deltoids	1-2	10-15
Prone back raise	Erector spinae	1-2	*
Trunk curl	Rectus abdominis	1-2	*

If desired, progress to 2 sets on selected exercises.

*Do as many repetitions as you can comfortably complete with body weight.

Table 9.3 Medicine Ball Exercises for Ages 7 to 10

Exercise	Muscle groups	Sets	Reps
Medicine ball front squat	Quadriceps Hamstrings Gluteals	1-2	10-15
Medicine ball lunge	Quadriceps Hamstrings Gluteals	1-2	10-15
Medicine ball supine chest press	Pectoralis major Front deltoid Triceps	1-2	10-15
Medicine ball pullover	Latissimus dorsi Deltoids	1-2	10-15
Medicine ball front shoulder raise	Deltoids	1-2	10-15
Medicine ball triceps press	Triceps	1-2	10-15
Medicine ball biceps curl	Biceps	1-2	10-15
Medicine ball curl-up	Rectus abdominis	1-2	10-15

If desired, progress to 2 sets on selected exercises.

competence and confidence in their ability to perform these movements with a wooden dowel, they progress to a lightweight aluminum barbell.

In physical education classes, it may be more feasible to develop a fitness circuit in which children travel around a gymnasium as they perform a series of strength-building exercises that are described on a poster at each station. A fitness circuit can include exercises with dumbbells, medicine balls, elastic bands, and body weight. By modifying the choice of the exercises as well as the duration of each activity, instructors can make strength training a safe, effective, and enjoyable activity for all children. For example, instead of beginning with body-weight exercises such as squats and zigzag jumps, children should start with relatively easy movements such as heel raises and jump-and-freeze drills. Children can exercise in groups of two or four as they move from station to station to complete the workout. Although competition among children is not the primary goal, keeping pace with others can add to the excitement of the class. This type of setup can foster participation and promote teamwork since each group must work together to be successful.

A sample fitness circuit with body-weight and medicine ball exercises for children is outlined in table 9.4. Note that some of the stations are modifications of exercises described in other chapters. For example, instead of a traditional push-up, which some young children have difficulty performing properly, station 1 is a push-up tap whereby a child starts in a push-up position and taps the chest with the hands as he maintains a rigid body position. The number of repetitions and time allotted at each station will vary depending on the fitness level of the participants and the time available for physical activity. In our elementary school programs, children spend 30 seconds at each station with a short rest interval (about 30 seconds) in between stations. Depending on the type of movement at each station, children typically perform 10 to 15 repetitions of each exercise. We use color-coded

Table 9.4 Fitness Circuit for Ages 7 to 10

Station 1: Push-up taps	Start in the push-up position. While maintaining a rigid body position, lift the right hand to tap the chest, then return the right hand to the floor. Repeat with the left hand and continue for the desired number of repetitions.
Station 2: Freezer jump	Jump as far forward as possible. Immediately upon landing, freeze and hold the position for a few seconds. Relax and then repeat.
Station 3: Elastic band biceps curl	Stand on top of a band with both feet while holding the ends of the band in each hand. Curl both hands upward toward the shoulders until your palms face your chest. Return to the starting position and repeat.
Station 4: Flutter feet	Start in the push-up position with both hands and both feet on the floor. While maintaining a stationary body position with both legs extended, lift the right foot off the floor a few inches and then return to the starting position. Repeat this flutter action with the left leg and continue alternating lifts for the desired number of repetitions.
Station 5: Single-leg reach	While balancing on the right foot, attempt to touch a ball or cone placed a few feet away by lowering the body and reaching forward with the left hand. Return to the starting position and repeat. Then perform the exercise while standing on the left foot and reaching with the right hand.
Station 6: High five	Stand about 3 feet (1 m) from a partner. Jump up and extend one arm as high as possible; attempt to touch your partner's hand while in the air. Land in a controlled manner and repeat.
Station 7: Standing partner twist	Stand back to back about 1 foot (0.3 m) from a partner. Pass a medicine ball back and forth by twisting the torso so the ball passes in front of the abdomen.
Station 8: Target practice	Toss a medicine ball into a hula hoop placed a few feet away. This activity does not require maximal effort but the ability to adjust muscular tension to achieve the desired result.
Station 9: Elastic band upright row	Stand on top of a band with both feet while holding the ends of the band in each hand with palms facing your body. Hold the band so that it hangs straight down in front of your body with your hands closer than shoulder-width apart. Pull the bands toward the chin while keeping both elbows pointing out to the sides; then lower the cord to the starting position and repeat.
Station 10: ABC ball	While holding a medicine ball with both hands, move the ball in various directions to draw large letters to spell a word or name.
Station 11: Ball crunch	Start in the sit-up position with both knees bent at a 90-degree angle. Lift both feet off the floor and place a medicine ball (or playground ball) on the shins. Lift the shoulder blades off the floor and touch the ball with both hands while keeping the lower back on the floor. Return to starting position and repeat.
Station 12: Walking lunge	Hold a medicine ball (or playground ball) against the chest with both hands. Take a long step forward with the right leg and then the left leg for the desired number of repetitions.

movement markers for each exercise, which make setting up a fitness circuit simple and efficient. You can make the fitness circuit more challenging by changing the choice of exercises, time at each station, rest interval between stations, or number of sets.

Training Considerations

Although body-weight exercises are an effective method of strength training, some 7- to 10-year-old children who are unfit or overweight may not be strong enough to do standard body-weight exercises, such as pull-ups, push-ups, and bar dips. In this case, modify the exercise or use machine, free-weight, or medicine ball exercises in which you can adjust the resistance

to each person's strength level. For example, an overweight child may not be able to perform a push-up but can complete 10 bench presses with 8-pound (3.5 kg) dumbbells or 15 repetitions of a medicine ball chest pass. Although all exercises address the same muscle groups (pectoralis major, front deltoid, triceps), 10 to 15 properly performed repetitions with dumbbells or medicine balls are obviously safer and more productive than struggling through a single push-up. As this child's upper-body strength improves, push-ups can be sensibly incorporated into the fitness program.

Of course, the key to safe and effective strength training is proper form, so instructors and coaches must focus on correct exercise technique at all times. Because some elastic-band exercises can be challenging, it is best to introduce this mode of training to children with relatively easy exercises such as the biceps curl or lateral raise and then progress to more advanced multijoint movements. Also, most children will prefer using 6-inch-wide (15 cm) elastic bands that can be cut to the desired length. As such, they will not need to wrap the ends of a long rubber tube around the wrists to ensure proper fit when performing an exercise.

Two things are essential in working with 7- to 10-year-old boys and girls: competent instruction and careful supervision. Teaching segments must be clear and concise, with brief explanations and perfect demonstrations, so that the youth can easily understand and model proper training technique. Even after the children have mastered the exercise technique, observe and interact with them as much as possible throughout each training session to reinforce their efforts and maintain their enthusiasm for the program. Attention to each participant is the top priority for safe and productive youth strength-training programs. Please note that you should never permit 7- to 10-year-old boys and girls to lift weights without appropriate supervision. This is especially true for at-home strength exercise, where a comfortable and familiar environment may reduce safety awareness and seriousness in training.

Sometimes it is necessary to modify an exercise by using tennis balls instead of dumbbells to ensure that a child can do the appropriate number of repetitions with the correct technique.

Teaching segments must be clear and concise, with brief explanations and perfect demonstrations, so that the youth can easily understand and model proper training technique.

Summary

Few physical activities offer as much opportunity for cooperation and mutual assistance as strength-training sessions. Teaching 7- to 10-year-olds to do sensible strength exercise is an educational endeavor that should have long-term benefits to health and fitness, especially for those who make strength training a standard component of their lives. Provided that qualified instruction is available, age 7 is not too young to experience and appreciate the benefits of supervised strength exercise. Just be sure to explain concepts at a level they understand, listen to individual concerns, and provide the instruction and attention necessary to ensure safe and successful training sessions. Finally, make every effort to emphasize the fun aspect of progressive strength training in order to spark a lifelong interest in physical activity.

10

INTERMEDIATE STRENGTH AND POWER FOR AGES 11 TO 14

Most of our youth strength-training studies have involved boys and girls in the 11- to 14-year-old range. These are ideal years to start a structured and carefully supervised program of resistance exercise. Throughout our two decades of youth strength-training experience, participants in this age group have consistently demonstrated high levels of interest, ability, and enthusiasm for strength-building exercise. They have also had excellent results, typically increasing their overall strength about 40 percent during the first two months of training. In addition, they have improved their body composition (more muscle and less fat), increased their self-confidence, and enhanced their sport performance.

Components of the Warm-Up and Cool-Down

Certainly, 11- to 14-year-olds should do other physical activities in addition to strength training. Although some program participants enjoy doing specific endurance exercises, such as bicycling or swimming, most boys and girls in this age range prefer a variety of movement activities in a game atmosphere. Therefore, have the children perform various locomotor skills before and after their training sessions. You may do

some dynamic warm-up activities with music and incorporate apparatus such as medicine balls, hoops, cones, steps, and elastic bands for challenge and variety. Be sure to include several static stretching exercises during the cool-down segments to enhance joint flexibility. Generally, a 45-minute session should consist of about 10 minutes of warm-up activity, 25 to 30 minutes of strength exercise, and 5 to 10 minutes of cool-down activity.

> Do some dynamic warm-up activities with music and incorporate apparatus such as medicine balls, hoops, cones, steps, and elastic bands for challenge and variety.

Strength-Training Program

Although some tall 11- to 14-year-olds fit adult-sized resistance machines, most preteens do better with free weights, medicine balls, or youth-sized weight machines. The National Strength and Conditioning Association's guidelines of one to three sets of 6 to 15 repetitions are appropriate for this age group, although our participants have had better results training in the 10- to

15-repetition range during the first few weeks of training. Because 11- to 14-year-olds attain similar results with two or three nonconsecutive exercise sessions per week, either of these training frequencies will be effective.

Depending on the exercises used, we recommend a program of 8 to 12 different strength exercises. A combination of multiple-muscle exercises, such as leg presses and bench presses, and single-muscle exercises, such as biceps curls and triceps press-downs, may be most effective in addressing all the major muscle groups. While it is easier to learn proper exercise technique on a weight machine that allows movement only in one plane or direction, it is important for youth to learn how to strength train using other types of equipment such as free weights and medicine balls. Since free weights and medicine balls require participants to balance the weight in all directions, other muscles besides the prime movers are activated. For example, the prime movers for the leg press exercise are the quadriceps, gluteals, and hamstrings, whereas the barbell squat exercise activates the same prime movers as well as secondary stabilizing muscles located on the upper body, lower body, and abdominal region.

A combination of multiple-muscle exercises, such as leg presses and bench presses, and single-muscle exercises, such as biceps curls and triceps press-downs, may be most effective in addressing all the major muscle groups.

In most strength-training classes for this age group, a combination of various types of training equipment will be most advantageous. Exercises on weight machines will provide an opportunity for less fit participants to gain confidence in their abilities to perform selected exercises while increasing the strength of specific muscle groups. Moreover, some exercises such as leg curls and front pull-downs require the use of a weight machine. On the other hand, since exercises performed with free weights and medicine balls can strengthen total-body movements and improve coordination, these movements might

better prepare preteens for activities of daily life and sports. Although a high degree of skill-related fitness is not a prerequisite for a lifetime of physical activity, confidence and competence in the ability to perform advanced exercises can indeed contribute to a child's health and well-being.

In our strength-training programs for youth ages 11 to 14, we use a combination of exercises that enhance muscular strength as well as other fundamental fitness abilities, including agility, balance, coordination, and power. We gradually progress from relatively simple exercises to more complex movements that require participants to think about what they are doing and how they are moving. For example, exercises such as the back squat and medicine ball lunge pass are cognitively stimulating movements that can result in real learning, provided that participants are taught how to perform these exercises with an appropriate load. In many instances, complex exercises that mimic natural body positions and movement speeds in daily life and game situations make strength training so valuable and enjoyable for this age group.

Machine Strength-Training Exercises

Table 10.1 presents sample strength exercises for 11- to 14-year-old boys and girls using youth-sized weight machines, along with recommendations for training sets, repetitions, and frequency. There are several types of weight machines, but the most important consideration is proper fit. Since the limbs of most preteens are too short for adult-sized weight machines, it is virtually impossible for these participants to

There are several types of weight machines, but the most important consideration is proper fit. Since the limbs of most preteens are too short for adult-sized weight machines, it is virtually impossible for these participants to safely perform the exercises through a full range of motion.

Table 10.1 Youth-Sized Machine Exercises for Ages 11 to 14

Exercise	Muscle groups	Sets	Reps
Leg press	Quadriceps Hamstrings Gluteals	1-3	10-15
Leg extension	Quadriceps	1-2	10-15
Leg curl	Hamstrings	1-2	10-15
Chest press	Pectoralis major Front deltoid Triceps	1-3	10-15
Front pull-down	Latissimus dorsi Rear deltoid Biceps	1-3	10-15
Overhead press	Deltoids Triceps Upper trapezius	1-2	10-15
Biceps curl	Biceps	1-2	10-15
Triceps press-down	Triceps	1-2	10-15
Hanging-knee raise	Hip flexors Rectus abdominis	1-2	10-15
Back extension	Erector spinae	1-2	10-15
Abdominal curl	Rectus abdominis	1-2	10-15

If desired, progress to 2 or 3 sets on selected exercises.

safely perform the exercises through a full range of motion. Thus, in most cases child-sized weight machines are more appropriate for preteens. Still, instructors and coaches should realize that a tall preteen or young teenager might be able to safely use adult-sized weight machines. By adjusting the seat or by using an additional back pad, a tall 12-year-old might be able to use selected adult-sized weight machines. In any case, always check each child for proper positioning of the arms and legs with the contact points on each weight machine. If a child of any age cannot properly fit onto a child- or adult-sized weight machine, that child should use another type of training equipment to strengthen those muscle groups.

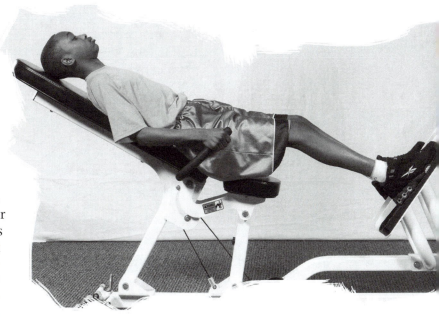

Make sure the child properly fits onto the weight machine to perform an exercise.

Free-Weight Strength-Training Exercises

Although weight machines offer many advantages, 11- to 14-year-old boys and girls can attain excellent results while training with free-weight equipment. Because proper fit is not a concern when using barbells and dumbbells, participants of various body sizes and experience can perform an unlimited number of exercises. We recommend beginning with a basic dumbbell program that includes both single-joint and multijoint exercises. Obviously, depending on the needs, goals, and abilities of the participants, you can modify this program by changing the exercises or the program variables. For example, if time is limited, participants can perform more multijoint exercises than single-joint exercises in order to efficiently train all the major muscle groups. Thus, boys and girls can learn how to perform new multijoint exercises with dumbbells or more advanced weightlifting movements with a wooden dowel or unloaded barbell. Participants who gain experience in their abilities to perform weightlifting movements during the preteen years will be able to perform these lifts with more confidence and competence during their teenage years. Table 10.2 presents sample strength exercises and training recommendations for 11- to 14-year-olds using dumbbells.

> Because proper fit is not a concern when using barbells and dumbbells, participants of various body sizes and experience can perform an unlimited number of exercises.

Medicine Ball Strength-Training Exercises

In addition to weight machines and free weights, medicine balls can safely strengthen all the major muscle groups. Medicine balls are versatile

Table 10.2   Dumbbell Exercises for Ages 11 to 14

Exercise	Muscle groups	Sets/reps	Reps
Dumbbell squat	Quadriceps Hamstrings Gluteals	1-3	10-15
Dumbbell bench press	Pectoralis major Front deltoid Triceps	1-3	10-15
Dumbbell one-arm row	Latissimus dorsi Rear deltoid Biceps	1-3	10-15
Dumbbell incline press	Deltoids Pectoralis major Triceps	1-2	10-15
Dumbbell biceps curl	Biceps	1-2	10-15
Dumbbell triceps kickback	Triceps	1-2	10-15
Prone back raise	Erector spinae	1-2*	10-15
Trunk curl	Rectus abdominis	1-2*	10-15

If desired, progress to 2 or 3 sets on selected exercises. Active supervision and spotting are important for preventing accidents and injuries.

*Do as many repetitions as you can comfortably complete with body weight.

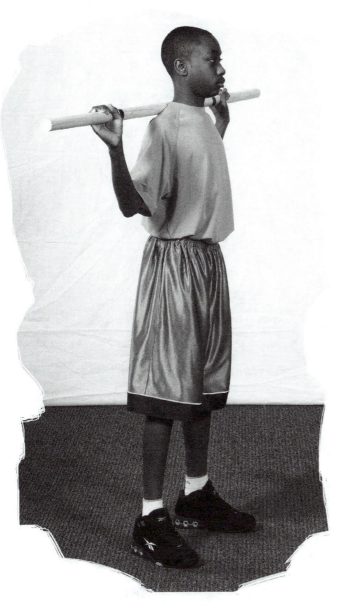

Children can learn proper exercise technique with a wooden dowel.

balls. Table 10.3 presents sample exercises and training recommendations for 11- to 14-year-olds using medicine balls. Note that participants should perform strength-training exercises for 10 to 15 repetitions, whereas they can do power exercises with medicine balls explosively for 6 to 8 repetitions.

Training Considerations

Some children in the 11- to 14-year-old age group are capable of doing body-weight exercises, such as push-ups and chin-ups. Those who participate in a progressive strength-training program should find it much easier to perform their body-weight exercises. You may include body-weight exercises in the overall conditioning program or use them exclusively if adjustable resistance exercises are not available. Keep in mind that the best way to build muscle strength is by gradually increasing the exercise resistance rather than simply adding more repetitions to fixed-weight movements.

Although push-ups are the standard upper-body exercise, bar dips provide an excellent alternative and address the same major muscles (chest, triceps, front shoulders) and place less stress on the lower back. However, heavy boys and girls who perform bar dips must make sure they do not descend too far or too fast. Other useful body-weight exercises are trunk curls and hanging-knee raises for the abdominal muscles and chin-up modifications for the upper-back and biceps muscles.

The weight-assisted chin-up and bar dip machines available in most fitness centers enable youth to perform body-weight exercises with less than their own body weight. For example, a boy who weighs 100 pounds and places 30 pounds on the weight stack actually lifts 70 pounds of his body weight on each chin-up or bar dip. As he becomes stronger, he may place less weight on the weight stack and use more of his own body weight. In this manner, all participants can perform these challenging exercises and progressively increase the resistance as they develop strength.

Participants in this age group may also work with elastic bands, because these children typically have sufficient coordination to stabilize their bodies as they perform the exercises. Children can perform a variety of single-joint and multi-joint exercises with elastic bands, and spotting is not normally required. However, since the

because they come in various shapes and sizes and can be used in gymnasiums and on playing fields. Participants can also perform partner exercises with medicine balls, which will keep them motivated. As with other types of strength training, it is important to learn proper exercise technique and start with a lightweight medicine ball and gradually progress. In some cases, medicine ball exercises can be incorporated into a dynamic warm-up or used for teaching more advanced exercises. For example, teachers and coaches can introduce participants to proper exercise technique for the squat or power clean by using 2.2- or 4.4-pound (1- or 2-kg) medicine

Table 10.3 Medicine Ball Exercises for Ages 11 to 14

Exercise	Muscle groups	Sets	Reps
Medicine ball squat toss	Quadriceps Hamstrings Gluteals	1-3	6-8
Medicine ball chest push	Pectoralis major Front deltoid Triceps	1-3	6-8
Medicine ball overhead throw	Latissimus dorsi Deltoids Triceps	1-3	6-8
Medicine ball front squat	Quadriceps Hamstrings Gluteals	1-3	10-15
Medicine ball walking lunge	Quadriceps Hamstrings Gluteals	1-2	10-15
Medicine ball single-leg dip	Quadriceps Hamstrings Gluteals	1-2	10-15
Medicine ball single-arm toss	Deltoids Triceps	1-2	10-15
Medicine ball lower- back lift	Erector spinae	1-2	10-15
Medicine ball twist and turn	Rectus abdominis Obliques	1-2	10-15
Medicine ball two-hand hold	Rectus abdominis Obliques	1-2	10-15 sec.

If desired, progress to 2 sets on selected exercises.

The weight-assisted chin-up and bar dip machines available in most fitness centers enable youth to perform body-weight exercises with less than their own body weight. For example, a boy who weighs 100 pounds and places 30 pounds on the weight stack actually lifts 70 pounds of his body weight on each chin-up or bar dip.

movement becomes more difficult as the band is stretched, instructors and coaches should ensure that participants perform each repetition in a controlled manner through the full range of motion. If exercise technique starts to falter during the middle or end of a repetition, the child should use a thinner band to allow for the proper completion of the exercise movement. Exercises with elastic bands can be incorporated into the warm-up period or the strength-training program.

As with younger boys and girls, the critical factors for safe and successful strength-training

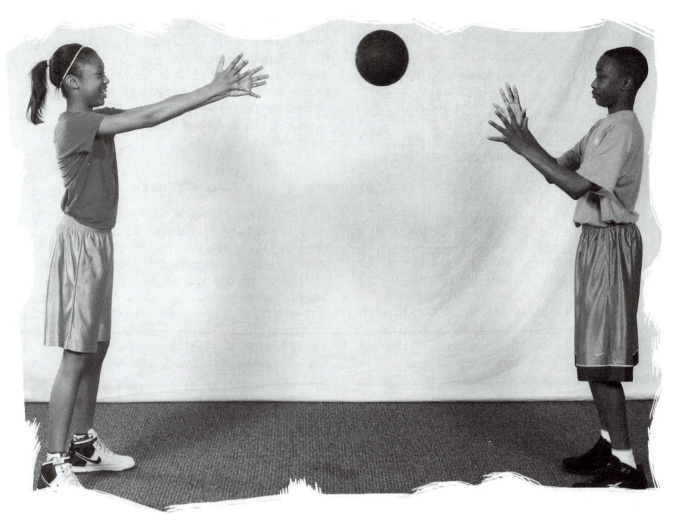

Medicine balls strengthen all major muscle groups.

experiences are competent instruction and careful supervision. Be sure to introduce each exercise with a concise explanation and precise demonstration. Follow up with careful observation and frequent interactions that include plenty of positive reinforcement for appropriate training behavior. Although 11- to 14-year-olds perform well in strength-training classes, do not permit them to exercise in unsupervised settings. In particular, they should do at-home strength training with parents or other adults who have experience with strength training in order to ensure proper exercise technique and safety awareness.

Most 11- to 14-year-old boys and girls are highly receptive and responsive to structured strength-training programs. While this type of strength training has proven to be effective, in some cases teachers and coaches might want to add variety to the program by creating a fitness circuit. Also, some teachers and coaches might not have access to weight machines and free weights and therefore need to be creative when developing their lesson plans. As described in chapter 9, developmentally appropriate fitness circuits can foster and encourage boys and girls of all abilities to participate in physical activity. You can use the fitness circuit described in chapter 9 and modify the program to make it more challenging for 11- to 14-year-old boys and girls. For example, participants can perform traditional push-ups instead of push-up taps and a medicine ball twist and turn instead of ball crunches.

Even if equipment is limited, teachers and coaches can create fitness circuits using body-weight exercises and a few medicine balls or elastic bands. Participants can travel around the gymnasium in groups of two to four as they perform a series of 8 to 12 exercises at various

Although 11- to 14-year-olds perform well in strength-training classes, do not permit them to exercise in unsupervised settings. In particular, they should do at-home strength training with parents or other adults who have experience with strength training in order to ensure proper exercise technique and safety awareness.

stations. The number of repetitions and time at each station will depend on the fitness level of the participants and the time allotted for physical activity, although 30 seconds at each station with a 30-second rest between stations is typically recommended. Most 11- to 14-year-old boys and girls respond favorably to circuit training and enjoy the experience of strength training with their friends. By exercising in an environment in which children feel socially safe, they will be more willing to try new exercises without fear of failure or public humiliation. In our youth programs, we give 11- to 14-year-olds a sense of control by allowing them to create new exercises that can be added to the fitness circuit. This experience teaches them self-responsibility and gives them a sense of control over the fitness circuit.

Summary

Children in this age range who perform strength exercises as part of a structured program or fitness circuit are likely to perform other physical activities and make healthy food selections. With clear objectives, age-appropriate exercises, sensible progression, and qualified instruction, strength training can be a worthwhile addition to any physical education or sport program. Every indication is that these are ideal years for introducing strength training for health, fitness, and sport.

11

ADVANCED STRENGTH AND POWER FOR AGES 15 TO 18

Although genetics clearly control the growth processes, teens who regularly perform strength exercises have certain developmental advantages over those who do not. Regular participation in a strength-training program increases musculoskeletal strength, improves body composition, and enhances the preparedness of aspiring young athletes for sport practice and competition. Clinical research and observations show that teens who participate in strength-training programs experience more favorable changes in muscle and strength development and are less likely to experience a sport-related injury. Furthermore, strength training is an activity that teens with varied needs, goals, and abilities can do with a partner or in small groups.

In our youth programs, we help teenagers develop the skills and knowledge that will lead to a lifetime of physical activity. While showing improvements on measures of physical fitness is important, we realize that educating teens about the importance of regular strength training is also important. Thus, we value the process of helping teens become self-directed as they develop good habits and plan their own fitness programs. Social support from teachers, parents, and peers; active participation in the design of the fitness program;

and personalized methods of monitoring progress can all help to promote regular physical activity in teenagers. In our youth program, participants monitor their progress on workout logs, and teens who have more experience strength training offer assistance and encouragement to those who are beginners. When appropriate, we also give teens a choice of exercises to enhance adherence.

Because physical appearance and athletic performance are valued characteristics among most teenagers, sensible strength training can be highly beneficial. On the other hand, teens who adhere to the high-volume exercise programs presented in popular muscle magazines tend to focus their training on selected muscle groups such as the biceps and chest. These programs can result in overtraining because they typically require dozens of exercises performed for several sets each. For these reasons, strength-training programs for teenagers must be carefully designed to address all major muscle groups with a reasonable number of exercises and moderate duration of workouts. Qualified instruction is essential for encouraging the adolescents who are less muscular and underconfident and for controlling those who are more muscular and overconfident.

Components of the Warm-Up and Cool-Down

Generally, teenagers are busy, with plenty of people to see, places to go, and things to do. For these reasons, teen strength-training sessions should be well designed, with little wasted time. Nevertheless, the warm-up and cool-down are still important and should be part of each strength-training session. To provide both muscular and cardiorespiratory conditioning in the overall training program, begin each 45-minute strength training session with a 10-minute dynamic warm-up that includes hops, skips, jumps, lunges, and various other movements for the upper and lower body. In addition to elevating core body temperature, this type of warm-up can improve mobility and prepare teens for strength-training activities. Teens are typically willing to perform a few static stretching exercises during the cool-down period, which typically lasts about 5 minutes, and this is the ideal time to enhance flexibility and recovery from the training session.

Strength-Training Program

Most 15- to 18-year-olds are large enough to train on adult-sized resistance machines, especially those that involve pushing or pulling movements such as the leg press, bench press, and seated row machines. They are also capable of executing most free-weight exercises properly and safely, given appropriate instruction and supervision. With careful spotting, teenagers may perform barbell bench presses and barbell squats as well as more advanced weightlifting movements. However, we strongly advise beginning these exercises with an unloaded barbell, plastic training plates, or even a wooden dowel until the participant develops proper technique. If you include these lifts in the training program, qualified teachers and coaches need to provide instruction and supervision.

Most 15- to 18-year-olds are large enough to train on adult-sized resistance machines, especially those that involve pushing or pulling movements such as the leg press, bench press, and seated row machines.

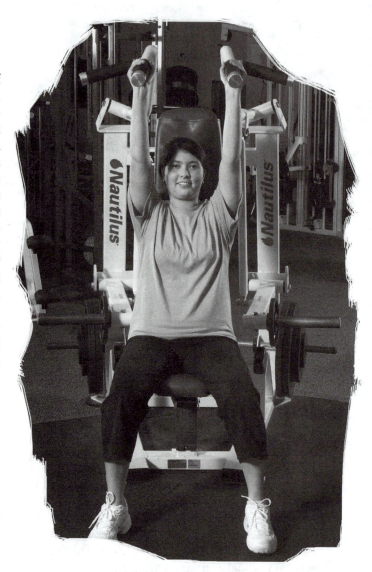

On a plate-loaded machine, each arm can move independently. It provides a combination of free weight and machine training.

Although weight machines offer safety advantages, some teens prefer equipment that uses barbell plates because each arm can move independently on this type of equipment. Plate-loaded equipment is durable and provides a user-friendly combination of free-weight and machine training. Of course, you must take care when loading and unloading the barbell plates. By enforcing the two-hand rule for carrying weight plates, you will greatly reduce the risk of injury from a dropped weight.

The National Strength and Conditioning Association recommends that teenagers perform training exercises for one to three sets of 6 to 15 repetitions each. Because of facilities, equipment availability, or philosophy, the number of exercises teens perform will vary, but generally 8 to 12 exercises for the upper body, lower body, and midsection are prescribed. Beginners may start with one set of 10 to 15 repetitions and progress to two or three sets of 8 to 12 repetitions after four to eight weeks of training. However, note that not all exercises need to be performed for the same number of sets. If the total training time is limited, consider performing one set on small-muscle-group exercises and multiple sets on large-muscle-group exercises. A training frequency of two or three times per week on nonconsecutive days is appropriate for most teens.

Generally, we characterize advanced training as more multiple-muscle free-weight exercises, extra sets, higher weight loads, and fewer repetitions than beginning exercise protocols. Typical single-joint machine exercises are the leg extension and leg curl, and typical multijoint free-weight exercises are the squat and bench press. Of course, there is nothing wrong with a workout that combines several single-joint and multijoint exercises. In most instances, a workout that consists of a variety of exercises tends to be the most effective and enjoyable. Once teens in our classes learn the basic skills, we give them a sense of control over the exercises by providing them with the opportunity to make decisions about the content of their workouts. This type of control allows teens to be creative and teaches them self-responsibility, which help them develop lifetime habits of physical activity.

Machine and Free-Weight Strength-Training Exercises

Although many combinations of productive free-weight and machine protocols are possible, tables 11.1 and 11.2 represent good starting points for overall muscle and strength development. Table 11.1 presents 12 basic free-weight exercises for 15- to 18-year-olds that address most major muscle groups. Teens who train with machines should attain good results with the 14-station program presented in table 11.2, provided that a variety of resistance machines are available. Teens involved in sports should also perform neck extensions and neck flexions to condition this vulnerable area of the body and thereby

reduce the risk of catastrophic injury. Since all modes of strength training have their advantages and disadvantages, the best approach may be to use a variety of training equipment to develop a well-rounded strength-training program.

> Since all modes of strength training have their advantages and disadvantages, the best approach may be to use a variety of training equipment to develop a well-rounded strength-training program.

Medicine Ball and Elastic Band Strength-Training Exercises

Participants in this age group can certainly train with medicine balls and elastic bands safely and effectively. This type of training may be useful in class settings or on the field for sport teams because balls and bands are portable and easy to use. Medicine balls and elastic bands are inexpensive, but it is important to have balls and bands of various sizes and resistances to accommodate each participant's abilities in various exercises. The many medicine ball and elastic band exercises described in other chapters can be structured in a way that is appropriate for all teens. When youth are able to perform these movements correctly, they can incorporate more advanced movements into their strength-training programs. Table 11.3 on page 198 presents sample exercises and training recommendations for 15- to 18-year-olds using medicine balls. Note that strength-training exercises should be performed for 10 to 15 repetitions, whereas power exercises should be performed explosively for fewer than 8 repetitions.

Depending on class time, lesson objectives, and each student's fitness abilities, instructors and coaches can modify their lesson plan in order to incorporate some type of medicine ball or elastic band training into each class. Since teaching teens about their bodies, improving health- and skill-related components of fitness, and exposing youth to a variety of physical activities are important lesson objectives, every session does not need to be devoted entirely to strength

Table 11.1   Free-Weight Exercises (12 Stations) for Ages 15 to 18

Exercise	Muscle groups	Sets	Reps
Barbell squat	Quadriceps Hamstrings Gluteals	1-3	8-12
Dumbbell step-up	Quadriceps Hamstrings Gluteals	1-2	8-12
Barbell bench press	Pectoralis major Front deltoid Triceps	1-3	8-12
Dumbbell chest fly	Pectoralis major	1-2	8-12
Dumbbell one-arm row	Latissimus dorsi Rear deltoid Biceps	1-3	8-12
Chin-up	Latissimus dorsi Rear deltoid Biceps	1-2	*
Dumbbell overhead press	Deltoids Triceps Upper trapezius	1-2	8-12
Dumbbell biceps curl	Biceps	1-2	8-12
Dumbbell triceps extension	Triceps	1-2	8-12
Bar dip	Pectoralis major Front deltoid Triceps	1-2	*
Prone back raise	Erector spinae	1-2	*
Trunk curl	Rectus abdominis	1-2	*

Begin with 1 or 2 sets of 10 to 15 repetitions before progressing to 2 or 3 sets of 8 to 12 repetitions.

*Do as many repetitions as you can comfortably complete with body weight.

training. For example, teachers and coaches can "activate" physical education classes and sport practice sessions by incorporating medicine ball training into the first 10 to 15 minutes of every lesson. During this time teens can perform a variety of medicine ball exercises that progress from simple to more complex. Or teachers and coaches can focus on developing upper- or lower-body strength with elastic bands. Regardless of the type of equipment used, remember that the goal

Regardless of the type of equipment used, remember that the goal of performing strength exercises at the start of each session is not to fatigue the participants but to prepare the participants for the demands of physical education class or sport practice.

Table 11.2 Resistance Machine Exercises (14 Stations) for Ages 15 to 18

Exercise	Muscle groups	Sets	Reps
Leg press	Quadriceps Hamstrings Gluteals	1-3	8-12
Leg extension	Quadriceps	1-2	8-12
Leg curl	Hamstrings	1-2	8-12
Hip adduction	Hip adductors	1-2	8-12
Hip abduction	Hip abductors	1-2	8-12
Chest press	Pectoralis major Front deltoid Triceps	1-3	8-12
Seated row	Latissimus dorsi Rear deltoid Biceps	1-3	8-12
Overhead press	Deltoids Triceps Upper trapezius	1-2	8-12
Biceps curl	Biceps	1-2	8-12
Triceps extension	Triceps	1-2	8-12
Weight-assisted chin-up	Latissimus dorsi Rear deltoid Biceps	1-2	8-12
Weight-assisted bar dip	Pectoralis major Front deltoid Triceps	1-2	8-12
Lower-back extension	Erector spinae	1-2	8-12
Abdominal curl	Rectus abdominis	1-2	8-12

Begin with 1 or 2 sets of 10 to 15 repetitions before progressing to 2 or 3 sets of 8 to 12 repetitions.

of performing strength exercises at the start of each session is not to fatigue the participants but to prepare the participants for the demands of physical education class or sport practice. Our program simply gives instructors a model from which they can use their own creativity and ideas to enhance the health and fitness of teens in their programs.

Training Considerations

The key to safe, effective, and enjoyable youth strength-training experiences is to develop a progressive program that is consistent with each participant's needs, goals, and abilities. With encouragement and support from adults and peers, teens will experience feelings of competence

Table 11.3 Medicine Ball Exercises for Ages 15 to 18

Exercise	Muscle groups	Sets	Reps
Medicine ball squat toss	Quadriceps Hamstrings Gluteals	1-3	6-8
Medicine ball lunge pass	Quadriceps Hamstrings Gluteals	1-3	6-8
Medicine ball chest pass	Pectoralis major Front deltoid Triceps	1-3	6-8
Medicine ball overhead throw	Latissimus dorsi Triceps Deltoids	1-3	6-8
Medicine ball backward throw	Latissimus dorsi Deltoids	1-2	6-8
Medicine ball side pass	Pectoralis major Front deltoid Triceps	1-2	6-8
Medicine ball overhead squat	Quadriceps Hamstrings Gluteals Deltoids	1-2	10-15
Medicine ball single-leg dip and reach	Quadriceps Hamstrings Gluteals Deltoids	1-2	10-15
Medicine ball push-up	Pectoralis major Front deltoid Triceps	1-2	10-15
Medicine ball lower-back lift	Erector spinae	1-2	10-15
Medicine ball V-sit	Rectus abdominis	1-2	10-15
Medicine ball twist and turn	Obliques	1-2	10-15

Begin with 1 or 2 sets before progressing to 3 sets on selected exercises.

and personal satisfaction. During every class, explain, demonstrate, then have the teens perform a new exercise while you provide constructive feedback. The goal is for all participants to develop good movement patterns characterized by proper exercise technique and movement speed. Once teens learn how to perform basic exercises, progress the program and add new exercises to spark their curiosity and challenge their physical skills. Without program variation and guidance from teachers and coaches, teens will likely become bored and frustrated.

Encourage teens to exercise with their peers and set realistic goals. Teach participants the concept of a fitness workout and reward the process of strength training rather than the product. Teachers and coaches must also provide an opportunity for all participants, not just teens who are naturally strong and fit, to feel good about strength training. For example, a 15-year-old girl who cannot lift her full body weight to perform a chin-up or bar dip should use weight-assisted chin-up and bar dip equipment if available to encourage a positive exercise experience. If this girl weighs 140 pounds, she could start with 70 pounds of body weight by placing 70 pounds on the weight stack. As she becomes stronger, she can train with 80 pounds of her body weight by placing 60 pounds on the weight stack. In other words, by systematically placing less weight on the weight stack, she can progressively increase her strength until she is capable of lifting her full body weight. The ability to handle body weight in chin-ups and bar dips typically increases a teen's self-confidence and provides positive reinforcement in their training efforts.

> Encourage teens to exercise with their peers and set realistic goals. Teach participants the concept of a fitness workout and reward the process of strength training rather than the product.

Although it is tempting to assume that athletic teens can attain high levels of muscular fitness through sport participation, that is seldom the case. In fact, to minimize risk of injury and maximize performance potential, aspiring young athletes should participate in strength-training programs that provide comprehensive muscle conditioning. In a growing number of cases, many teens are poorly prepared for the demands of both sport practice and competition. Clearly, a youngster's participation in sport should not start with competition but should evolve out of preparatory strength training and instructional practice sessions that are gradually progressed over time. In our youth sport programs, aspiring athletes participate in 6 to 8 weeks of preparatory strength training before sport participation. The training protocols pre-

sented in this chapter address all major muscle groups in a balanced manner and are appropriate for all teens. The sport-specific programs described in chapter 12 address the needs of young athletes.

After receiving proper exercise instruction and demonstrating ideal training technique, most teens can function independently in supervised fitness centers. Even under supervised conditions, however, it may be necessary to remind teens of safe and sensible strength-training procedures. Young teens should not compromise their exercise form under any circumstances. In

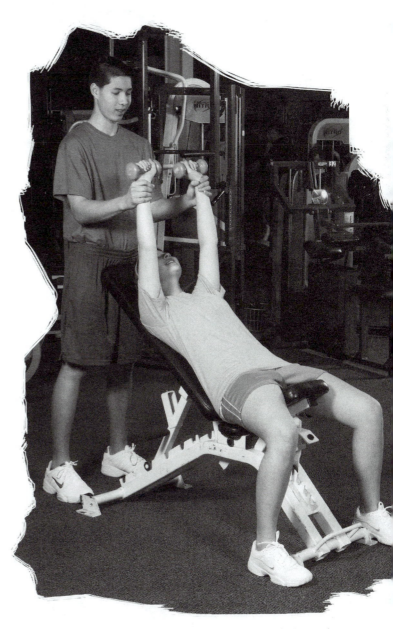

Encouragement and support from peers gives youth feelings of competence and satisfaction.

our strength-training programs, success is not measured simply by assessing gains in muscular strength but rather by mastering tasks and moving forward in difficulty levels.

Summary

Since teens who enjoy strength training are likely to become adults who get pleasure from this type of exercise, it is important to address individual needs, goals, and abilities when designing youth strength-training programs. Strength training may become a lifetime physical activity if teens experience feelings of confidence and personal satisfaction when training. A common goal for all teens is to develop good movement patterns on a variety of exercises. With qualified exercise instruction and program variation, teenagers will understand the concept of a fitness workout and will learn how to design and modify their own strength-training programs.

SPORT-SPECIFIC STRENGTH AND POWER FOR YOUNG ATHLETES

The number of children and adolescents involved in school-sponsored and community-based sport programs continues to increase. Although this is a favorable trend, in a growing number of cases the musculoskeletal systems of young athletes are not prepared for the demands of both sport practice and competition. Sport-related injuries are a significant cause of hospitalization and high health care costs during childhood and adolescence, and it is possible that certain youth sport injuries can increase the risk of osteoarthritis later in life. By addressing risk factors associated with youth sport injuries, some sports medicine physicians believe that both acute and overuse injuries could be significantly reduced by 15 to 50 percent. Research findings clearly illustrate the importance of strength training for safe and productive sport experiences.

Although each sport has unique conditioning requirements, young athletes should complete a general muscle-conditioning program before beginning a sport-specific strength and conditioning program. Not only will this provide them with an opportunity to improve their exercise technique, but if youth first enhance their strength in all the major muscle groups, they will be better prepared for more advanced training as well. On the other hand, if participants address only those muscles used in a particular sport or athletic event, those muscles are more likely to suffer overuse injuries, and the untrained muscles are more prone to traumatic injuries. In some cases, young athletes might need to reduce the amount of time they spend practicing sport-specific skills to allow time for preparatory strength and conditioning.

Even though youth who participate in recreational sports seem to have higher levels of strength and power than less active youth, it is unlikely that a child will gain the specific benefits of strength training without actually participating in a progressive strength-training program. Thus, it is prudent for all youth athletes to participate in well-designed strength-training programs that vary in volume and intensity throughout the year. This type of conditioning could enhance athletic performance and decrease the likelihood that youth drop out of sport because of frustration, embarrassment, failure, or injury. Regular strength training has proven to be particularly beneficial for young female athletes who appear to be more susceptible to knee injuries than young male athletes.

However, strength training should not simply be added into a young athlete's exercise regimen that already includes several hours of sport training and free play. A downfall of some youth strength-training programs is that adequate time

201

isn't allowed for recovery between training sessions. Because young athletes are still growing and developing, it is likely that they need even more time for rest and recovery between exercise sessions than adults do. Coaches who work with young athletes need to pay special attention to the intensity and volume of the exercise program as well as the amount of rest and recovery between exercise sessions if performance enhancement and injury reduction are primary training objectives. Modifying the design of the workout or changing the training frequency in response to a participant's ability (or inability) to respond to a strength-training program is vital for long-term success.

Training for Sport Conditioning

Successful sport performance requires a combination of strength, power, endurance, speed, agility, balance, and coordination. Although most conditioning programs for young athletes highlight the importance of specific strength-building exercises, don't overlook the value of power training, which requires the ability to achieve a high velocity while controlling a body position. Although strength training can make muscles stronger, power training can develop explosiveness and speed.

Weightlifting movements, plyometrics, and medicine ball exercises are ideal for power training because these exercises are performed quickly. In a power exercise, every repetition should be performed explosively without undue fatigue. Thus, youth should focus on increasing the speed of each movement, the height of each jump, or the distance they throw a ball. As youth gain confidence in their ability to perform these movements explosively, they can perform additional sets and repetitions, provided that they don't sacrifice movement quality. Moreover, to generate near-maximal power during the workout, participants should perform power exercises early in the workout before the strength exercises. With qualified coaching and a careful prescription of the program variables, power training can be safe, challenging, and fun.

Generally, power- and strength-training protocols should be effective with 1 to 3 sets per exercise. On the power exercises, use 6 to 8 repetitions per set, and work on increasing the speed of the exercise movement before you increase the weight or number of sets. On the strength-building exercises, repetition ranges should progress from higher to lower as muscle strength increases. Begin with 10 to 15 repetitions per set, then use more resistance for 8 to 10 repetitions, and then use 6 to 8 repetitions per set. Of course, not all exercises need to be performed for the same number of sets and repetitions. As a general guideline, all sport conditioning workouts should begin with dynamic warm-up activities and finish with cool-down activities that include static stretching.

In addition to sport-specific exercises for the major muscle groups, all workouts for athletes should include exercises that strengthen the abdominal and lower-back region. Not only is this area prone to injury, but the trunk region is also responsible for maintaining stability of the spine and transferring energy from large to small body parts during most sporting events. Strengthening the abdominal and lower-back region will enhance power production because movement will be more efficient. In addition to traditional exercises such as trunk curls and pelvic tilts, more advanced multidirectional exercises that involve rotational movements and diagonal patterns, performed with one's own body weight or a medicine ball, can be used in strengthening this area. Since movement in sport occurs in various plans of action, young athletes should perform a variety of exercises to strengthen their abdominal and lower-back musculature.

Although young sport participants may train three days per week during the off-season, they should cut back to two workouts per week during the in-season. The rigors of sport activity might make it difficult to achieve full muscle recovery when a child does demanding strength exercises every other day. Our research clearly shows that two training sessions per week produce almost as much gain in strength and muscle development as three weekly workouts. Sport coaches should be present and actively involved in each training session. It is important to encourage good training effort, ensure correct exercise technique, and reinforce appropriate attitudes and actions in the weight room.

Keep in mind that the suggested sport-specific exercise programs outlined in this chapter are not rigid guidelines, and coaches should modify them for each athlete and training circumstance. For example, during the off-season the focus of the program might be on enhancing strength and hypertrophy, whereas during the preseason the goal of the program might be to increase power. Thus, athletes might perform more strength-building exercises during the off-season and more power-training exercises during the preseason. Whatever the case might be, coaches should periodically vary the training program by systematically changing the exercises, sets, and repetitions in order to keep the training program effective. Additional information on program variation and periodization is discussed in chapter 13.

> Coaches should periodically vary the training program by systematically changing the exercises, sets, and repetitions in order to keep the training program effective.

The following programs present sport-specific training protocols that supplement general strength- and power-conditioning programs. Feel free to add, omit, or substitute exercises as necessary because of time constraints, equipment availability, conditioning objectives, and individual needs. While a comprehensive muscle-conditioning program is essential for successful athletic experiences, it is also important to guard against too much specialization early in a young athlete's career. Thus, the programs in this chapter address the specific needs of popular sports while strengthening all the major muscle groups. We group these training protocols according to the major emphasis of popular youth sports and activities.

Baseball and Softball

The sports of baseball and softball have many similarities, mostly related to inherent movement patterns. For example, baseball and softball share the component of striking a ball and require sprinting ability to run the bases. Power production for all striking actions is generated by the large muscles of the legs and hips, transferred through the rotational muscles of the midsection, accelerated by the shoulder muscles, and applied to the striking implement through the arms. Perfectly synchronized and properly executed striking actions are the result of a highly coordinated and complex series of movements that build on one another to maximize force output and swinging speed. Power exercises with medicine balls and movements that require rotation are appropriate for young athletes who participate in striking sports.

Because striking actions involve so many muscles, we suggest performing exercises that use two or more of the target muscle groups. These power- and strength-building exercises are consistent with the muscle actions and movements performed by baseball and softball players.

Baseball and Softball Sample Workout
Power skipping
Lateral jump
Medicine ball chest pass
Medicine ball overhead pass
Medicine ball side pass
Back squat or leg press
Leg curl
Heel raise
Bench press
Dumbbell row
Medicine ball push-up
Shoulder internal and external rotation
Wrist curl and extension (or wrist roller)
Lower-back exercises
Abdominal exercises

Basketball and Volleyball

A general strength and conditioning program should establish an excellent base from which to enhance jumping ability in basketball and volleyball. Nonetheless, sports that require plenty of powerful jumps can benefit from specialized training and specific power and strength exercises. For power development in the lower extremities, use weightlifting movements, plyometrics, and medicine ball exercises. These activities condition the legs to perform quickly and explosively. Although there are some differences in the jumping actions involved in basketball and volleyball, athletes use the same major muscle groups in all vertical jumps. Both single-leg and double-leg takeoffs are powered by the calf muscles of the lower leg, the quadriceps and hamstring muscles of the thigh, and the gluteal muscles of the hip. In addition to power exercise, strength-building exercises such as the squat and heel raise should provide plenty of conditioning for the quadriceps and calf muscles. The shoulder muscles (deltoids) also contribute to the jumping action by producing a powerful upward thrust, which is important in two-foot takeoffs.

Basketball and Volleyball Sample Workout

Ankle jumps

Standing jump and reach

90-degree jumps

Medicine ball chest pass

Medicine ball overhead pass

Power clean or power snatch

Push press

Back squat or leg press

Leg curl

Heel raise

Bench press

Front pull-down

Lower-back exercises

Abdominal exercises

Dancing and Figure Skating

Although there are obvious differences between jumping in a dance studio and jumping in an ice rink, the movement patterns and muscle actions are similar. Dancers and figure skaters can benefit by performing some targeted exercises that directly condition the major muscle groups that contribute most to jumping power. In addition, strengthening exercises for the hip adductors and hip abductors are important because inner- and outer-thigh muscles participate in the numerous lateral movements that characterize most dance and figure-skating performances. Most figure-skating jumps and many dance moves require midair turns that athletes accomplish using the midsection and shoulder muscles. Thus, exercises that strengthen the oblique muscles on the sides of the midsection should also be included in the workout.

Dancing and Figure Skating Sample Workout

Jump and freeze

90-degree jumps

Medicine ball lunge pass

Medicine ball side pass

Dumbbell squat or leg press

Hip abduction

Hip adduction

Heel raise

Dumbbell chest press

Dumbbell row

Lower-back exercises

Abdominal exercises

Football and Rugby

Participants in football and rugby should be well prepared for successful sport performance by following a progressive strength and conditioning program. Although the requirements for each position vary, these sports use muscles of the legs, chest, and arms in a pronounced pushing action. For power development, weightlifting movements, plyometrics, and medicine ball drills have proven to be effective for these athletes. For example, sprinting and blocking depend on leg strength and power, which can be enhanced by performing power cleans and push presses along with strength-building squats and heel raises. Because of the potential for catastrophic injury to the neck, it is essential to condition the neck muscles of young football and rugby players. In addition, these athletes should perform strengthening exercises for the lower back and rotator cuff because these are areas that are prone to injury.

Football and Rugby Sample Workout

Jump and freeze

Lateral cone jumps

Medicine ball squat toss

Medicine ball chest pass

Power clean

Push press

Back squat or leg press

Deadlift

Bench press

Seated row

Neck flexion and extension or shrugs

Internal and external shoulder rotation

Lower-back exercises

Abdominal exercises

Ice Hockey and Field Hockey

The striking actions in ice hockey and field hockey have many similarities and involve the same muscle groups for power production. Vertical striking movements derive most of their force from the large muscles of the legs and hips. As with horizontal swings, the powerful hip thrust that shifts weight from the rear leg to the front leg initiates the striking action. Although there is plenty of involvement from the quadriceps, hamstring, and gluteals, the hip adductor and hip abductor muscles of the inner and outer thigh are largely responsible for the rapid weight transfer and force development. The strength-training program should therefore include hip adduction and hip abduction exercises or side lunges with dumbbells to address these muscle groups.

Power generated in the lower body must pass to the upper body as efficiently as possible. The torquing action of the midsection muscles accomplishes and accelerates this. The lower back and abdominals contribute to the force transfer, but the oblique muscles on the sides of the midsection are key players in this phase of the swing. Also, strong forearm muscles ensure a secure yet relaxed grip on the stick and therefore enhance control of the striking implement.

Ice Hockey and Field Hockey Sample Workout

Lateral cone jumps

Zigzag jumps

Medicine ball lunge pass

Medicine ball side pass

Power clean

Back squat or leg press

Hip abductor

Hip adductor

Bench press

Seated row

Shoulder internal and external rotation

Wrist curl and extension (or wrist roller)

Lower-back exercises

Abdominal exercises

Soccer

Soccer is an endurance sport and, with the exception of goaltenders, athletes in this sport are usually constantly in motion. The continual action requires high levels of cardiorespiratory and muscular endurance for successful and sustained performance. Although soccer is less dependent on muscle strength than power sports, strength training should be a major component in the conditioning programs. First, because every physical action such as sprinting requires muscle strength, a stronger athlete has an advantage over a weaker athlete. This is especially true in soccer, which is characterized by stop-and-go activity and requires intermittent acceleration and deceleration. Second, because of the repetitive nature of soccer, these athletes have a high incidence of overuse injuries. Strength training improves muscle balance and increases musculoskeletal resistance to repetitive stress. Because soccer involves many lateral movements, the recommended training program addresses the muscles of the inner and outer thigh. Although upper-body strength might not be as important as lower-body strength, soccer players can benefit from a well-conditioned upper body.

Soccer Sample Workout

Lateral cone jumps

90-degree jumps

Power skipping

Medicine ball overhead pass

Dumbbell squat or leg press

Hip abductor

Hip adductor

Dumbbell chest press

Dumbbell row

Neck flexion and extension or shrugs

Lower-back exercises

Abdominal exercises

Swimming

Although swimming includes a variety of events from short to long duration, all swimmers can benefit from strength and power training. In addition to improving swim performance, swimmers can also reduce their risk of overuse injuries by developing balanced strength, especially around the shoulder joint. Because every swimming stroke requires a certain percentage of maximum strength, a stronger swimmer is definitely a better swimmer. An analysis of the muscles most relevant to swimming performance shows that the primary force producers for the arm-pulling action are the upper-back (latissimus dorsi) muscles. The chest (pectoralis major) and triceps muscles also contribute to pulling power. The shoulder (deltoid) muscles are most active during the recovery phase of the arm stroke, when the hand is out of the water. The leg action for flutter kicking is largely produced by the quadriceps, hamstrings, and gluteal muscles. Of course, breaststrokers should also perform hip adduction and hip abduction exercises for the inner- and outer-thigh muscles that are prominent in this swimming event. Because of the high incidence of rotator cuff injuries among swimmers, their strength-training program should include external and internal rotation exercises for the shoulders.

Swimming Sample Workout

Jump and freeze

Cone jumps

Medicine ball overhead pass

Medicine ball backward toss

Back squat or leg press

Bench press

Front pull-down

Dumbbell row

Medicine ball push-up

Lateral raise

Shoulder internal and external rotation

Triceps kickback

Lower-back exercises

Abdominal exercises

Tennis

The striking actions in tennis drives (forehand and backhand) are similar to those of other striking sports and derive power from essentially the same muscle groups. All horizontal striking movements are initiated by the large muscles of the legs and hips and are characterized by a powerful hip thrust that transfers weight from the rear leg to the front leg. Although most leg muscles contribute to this explosive action, the midsection, chest, and triceps are key players. It is also important to focus on developing forearm strength for gripping as well as muscle balance since one side of the body can dominate in tennis. Because of the potential for injury to the rotator cuff muscles and lower back, strengthening exercises for these muscle groups should also be included in the workout.

Tennis Sample Workout

Square jumps

90-degree jumps

Medicine ball lunge pass

Medicine ball side pass

Back squat or leg press

Dumbbell side lunge (or hip abduction and hip adduction)

Heel raises

Dumbbell chest press

Dumbbell row

Medicine ball push-up

Triceps kickback

Shoulder internal and external rotation

Wrist curl and extension (or wrist roller)

Lower-back exercises

Abdominal exercises

Track: Sprints and Jumps

Sprinting and jumping are powerful activities that can benefit from specialized training. Plyometric and medicine ball exercises for greater upper- and lower-body power and strength exercises for total-body conditioning have proven to be effective for these athletes. Every running stride is counterbalanced by a matching arm action, so the left leg and right arm always move in a synchronized pattern, as do the right leg and left arm. A strong upper body is therefore a great advantage when the legs start to tire, because an unrelenting arm drive will keep the legs moving in matching rhythm. Another important conditioning concern for sprinters and jumpers is the upper-back and shoulder area. For midsection conditioning, make sure every workout includes exercises that strengthen the oblique muscles that surround the sides and the lower back.

Sprints and Jumps Sample Workout

Ankle jumps

Cone jumps

Power skipping

Medicine ball squat toss

Medicine ball lunge pass

Power clean

Back squat or leg press

Leg curl

Heel raise

Bench press

Dumbbell row

Shoulder press

Lower-back exercises

Abdominal exercises

Track: Distance Running

Although distance runners and cross-country runners and are not power athletes, they can benefit from an appropriate strength and conditioning program. Perhaps the major advantage for strength-trained distance runners is the reduced risk of overuse injuries so prevalent in this sport. For example, since so many runners experience lower-leg injuries such as shin splints and stress fractures, it is beneficial to include a strengthening exercise for the shin muscles in order to maintain muscle balance in the lower leg. It is also advisable for runners to do

strengthening exercises for the abdominal and oblique muscles as well as for the upper-back and shoulder area. When this part of the body begins to fatigue and tighten up, the race is over. Training all major muscle groups to a high level of strength and muscular endurance ensures balanced muscle development and greater ability to absorb shock.

Distance Running Sample Workout

Medicine ball lunge pass

Medicine ball side pass

Leg press

Leg curl

Heel raise

Toe raise

Bench press

Seated row

Lateral raise

Lower-back exercises

Abdominal exercises

Summary

Regular participation in a strength-training program can enhance sport performance and reduce the likelihood of sport-related injuries. However, to be safe and effective, training programs need to be consistent with individual abilities, and young athletes need adequate time for rest and recovery between workouts. With qualified coaching and supervision, young athletes will look forward to strength and power training. Keep in mind that good coaching is as important in the weight room as on the athletic field. Competent instruction, positive reinforcement, and program variation are key factors in successful strength-training experiences.

PART IV

LONG-TERM PLANNING AND NUTRITIONAL SUPPORT

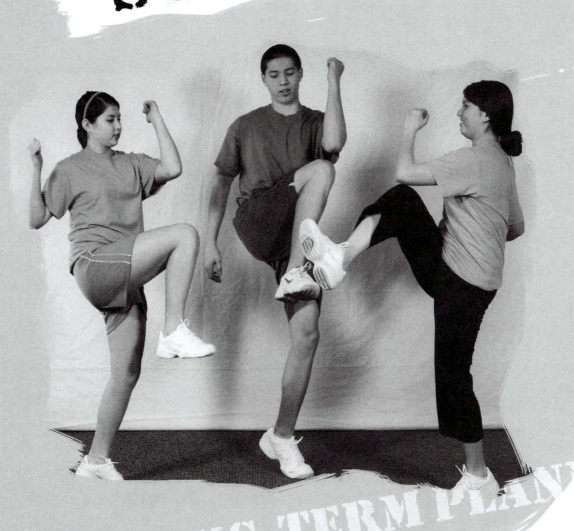

13

PERIODIZATION AND RECOVERY

The concept of program progression and long-term planning is known as periodization. Since it is impossible for children and teenagers to continually improve at the same rate over long-time periods, properly varying the training variables can limit training plateaus, maximize performance gains, and reduce the likelihood of overtraining. The underlying concept of periodization is based on Hans Selye's general adaptation syndrome, which proposes that after a period of time, adaptations to a new stimulus will no longer take place unless the stimulus is altered. Selye was an endocrinologist whose research on the role of stress hormones in the adaptation to stress provided the theoretical framework for periodization. Periodization is a process whereby instructors and coaches regularly change the training program in order to keep it effective and enjoyable. While the concept of periodization has been part of adult sport-training programs for many years, our understanding of the benefits of periodization and its application to youth has only recently been explored in the literature.

Periodization is not just for young athletes but also for children and teenagers with varying levels of training experience who want to enhance their health and fitness. By periodically changing program variables such as the choice of exercise, training weight (resistance), number of sets, rest periods between sets, or any combination of these, long-term performance gains will be optimized and the risk of overuse injuries will be reduced. Moreover, it is reasonable to suggest that youth who participate in well-designed periodized programs and continue to improve their health, fitness, and sport performance will be more likely to adhere to an exercise program for the long term.

For example, if a teenager's lower-body routine typically consists of the leg press, leg extension, and leg curl exercises, performing the dumbbell lunge, hip abduction, and hip adduction exercises on alternate workout days might increase the effectiveness of the training program and reduce the likelihood of staleness and boredom. Furthermore, varying the training weights, repetitions, number of sets, and rest interval between sets and exercises can help to prevent training plateaus, which are not uncommon in high school fitness centers. Many times a participant can avoid a strength plateau by decreasing the training intensity and training volume to allow for ample recovery. In the long term, program variation with adequate recovery will allow participants to attain higher strength levels because the body will be prepared to adapt to even greater demands. Periodization, which includes periods of reduced training, can optimize performance by keeping the training stimulus fresh and effective (see figure 13.1).

While untrained youth respond favorably to most reasonable strength-training protocols, trained individuals improve at a slower rate and require more advanced training programs

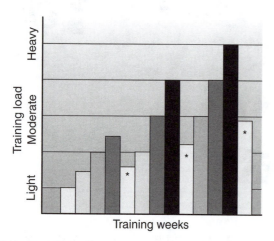

Figure 13.1 Program progression with less intense training periods* will optimize long-term adaptations.

in order to further enhance muscular strength. Thus, strength-training programs designed for beginners may not be effective for trained participants who have at least three months of strength-training experience. Clearly, there is not one model of strength exercise that will optimize training-induced adaptations in both untrained and trained people. Therefore, it is reasonable for beginners to start with a general strength-training program and gradually progress to more advanced training programs as performance and confidence improve. Since long-term progression in strength exercise requires a systematic manipulation of the program variables, teachers and coaches need to make important decisions regarding the exercise prescription. This requires a solid understanding of training-induced adaptations that take place in both beginners and experienced strength trainers. While limited variation is needed in beginners, as the program progresses more variation and more complex training regimens are needed.

Overreaching and Overtraining

Teachers and coaches need to balance the demands of training with adequate recovery between workouts in order to optimize training adaptations. A strength-training program characterized by an excessive frequency, volume, or intensity of training combined with inadequate rest and recovery will eventually result in over-training syndrome, which can ruin an athletic

career. In essence, overtraining syndrome might occur when the training stimulus exceeds the rate of adaptation. Overtraining syndrome typically includes a plateau or decrease in performance. Other observable manifestations of overtraining include decreased body weight, loss of appetite, sleep disturbances, decreased desire to train, muscle tenderness, and increased risk of infection.

> A strength-training program characterized by an excessive frequency, volume, or intensity of training combined with inadequate rest and recovery will eventually result in overtraining syndrome, which can ruin an athletic career.

For example, if a 12-year-old girl strength trains on Monday, Wednesday, and Friday and jogs on Tuesday, Thursday, and Saturday, the chronic forces placed on the lower body can injure muscles and connective tissue and decrease performance in the weight room and on the track. Overtraining can result from exercise programming characterized by frequent training sessions without adequate rest and recovery between workouts. From a practical perspective, it is important to consider each person's training experience as well as all the fitness activities regularly performed. Periodization can help to avoid overtraining and promote long-term gains in muscular fitness.

Overtraining on a short-term basis has become known as overreaching. Unlike recovery from overtraining syndrome, which can last for months, recovery from overreaching can occur within a few days. In fact, overreaching is sometimes a planned part of conditioning programs for athletes as well as recreational lifters who train at higher volumes and intensities. Nevertheless, overreaching should be considered the first stage of overtraining and therefore warrants attention because not all participants recover quickly from overreaching. Throughout every training program or sport season, youth will need to periodically decrease the intensity and volume of their workouts in order to allow time for recovery and a rebound in performance. In any case, it is always better to undertrain a young athlete than to overestimate his or her physical abilities and risk injury, illness, or burnout.

Models of Periodization

Although there are many models of periodization, the general concept is to prioritize training goals and then develop a long-term plan that varies throughout the year. In general, the year can be divided into specific training cycles with a specific goal for each cycle. A variety of exercises and combinations of sets and repetitions can optimize gains in strength or power. The classic model of periodization is referred to as a linear model because the volume and intensity of training gradually change over time. For example, at the start of the general preparation phase, the focus is on developing proper exercise technique with a light to moderate load in order to build a solid foundation for future conditioning. As the training progresses over time, the intensity of training increases in order to optimize gains in strength and power. Although participants progress at different rates, the general idea is to systematically modify the progression plan every two months or so in order to keep the program effective.

Although this type of periodized training originally was designed for adult athletes who attempted to peak for a competition, instructors and coaches can modify this model to enhance health and fitness in school-age youth. For example, children who routinely perform the same combination of sets and repetitions on all exercises can benefit from gradually increasing the weight and decreasing the number of rep-

etitions as strength improves. An example of a linear periodized plan, which consists of three distinct phases, is outlined in table 13.1. Note that the repetition maximum, or RM load, gradually progresses from a weight that can be lifted for not more than 15 repetitions to a heavier load that can be lifted for 8 repetitions or fewer. Since it is not possible to maintain peak levels of strength and power for a prolonged period, this model of training allows young athletes to adapt to various training protocols while reaching peak condition at the appropriate time. Obviously, when designing any youth strength-training program, coaches and instructors have to consider the specific requirements of an athlete's sport as well as individual needs, goals, and abilities of that athlete.

> Since it is not possible to maintain peak levels of strength and power for a prolonged period, the linear model of training allows young athletes to adapt to various training protocols while reaching peak condition at the appropriate time.

After the three-phase program is complete, participants should be encouraged to participate in recreational activities or low-intensity resistance training to reduce the likelihood of overtraining. This period of restoration is referred to as active rest and typically lasts for one to two weeks. Teachers and coaches may find it worthwhile to consider a youngster's academic schedule or vacation plans when incorporating

Table 13.1   Sample Linear Periodized Strength-Training Workout

	Phase 1: general preparation	Phase 2: strength	Phase 3: power
Intensity	10- to 15RM	8- to 10RM	6- to 8RM
Sets	1-2	2-3	3
Rest period between sets and exercises	1 min.	1-2 min.	2 min.

This plan is for the exercises of the major muscle groups performed in each phase. RM = repetition maximum. Phases 1, 2, and 3 last about 2 months each.

periods of active rest into a yearlong training schedule. After active rest, participants can then return to phase 1 of the training program with more energy and vigor.

A second model of periodization is referred to as an undulating (nonlinear) model because of the daily fluctuations in training volume and intensity. For example, on the major exercises for the legs, chest, and back, a person might perform two sets of 10 to 12 repetitions with a moderate load on Monday, three sets of 6 to 8 repetitions with a heavier load on Wednesday, and one set of 13 to 15 repetitions with a lighter load on Friday. Whereas the heavy training days will maximally activate the trained musculature, selected muscle fibers will not be maximally taxed on light and moderate training days. By alternating training intensities, the participant can minimize the risk of overtraining and maximize the potential for maintaining training-induced strength gains. A sample nonlinear periodized workout plan is presented in table 13.2. Every two to three months, periods of active rest lasting from one to two weeks will allow for physical and psychological recovery from the strength-training sessions.

Rest and Recovery

While more has been written about how to design strength-training programs than how to recover from practice and training, working with youth of any age involves balancing the demands of training (required for adaptation) with recovery (also required for adaptation). Although some parents, teachers, and coaches still have a "more is better" attitude, the perception that boys and girls can recover from hard workouts faster than adults is not supported by research.

Since children and adolescents are still growing and developing, we believe that youth may actually need more time than adults for recovery between high-volume and high-intensity training sessions. Although a day off between workouts might be adequate for youth who participate in recreational strength-training programs, training to enhance sport performance involves higher levels of physical as well as psychological stress. Therefore, well-planned activities are needed in order to maximize recovery and return to an optimal performance state. Thus, appropriate recovery is particularly important for youth who participate in more than one sport, specialize in one sport year round, or participate in extracurricular strength and conditioning activities.

Although some parents, teachers, and coaches still have a "more is better" attitude, the perception that boys and girls can recover from hard workouts faster than adults is not supported by research.

Since recovery is an integral part of any child's training program, we incorporate less intense training, or LIT, sessions into our youth programs as part of our periodized training cycle. Instead of simply taking a day off, our participants have LIT sessions that include activities that facilitate recovery, enhance joint stability, improve range of motion, and reinforce learning of specific movement patterns. LIT sessions are valued by our young participants as an important component of our multifaceted approach to enhancing performance and optimizing recovery. Since the greatest adaptations take place

Table 13.2 Sample Nonlinear Periodized Strength-Training Workout

	Monday	Wednesday	Friday
Intensity (RM)	10- to 12RM	6- to 8RM	13- to 15RM
Sets	2	3	1
Rest period between sets and exercises	1-2 min.	2 min.	1 min.

This plan is for the exercises of the major muscle groups performed each day. RM = repetition maximum.

when the muscles have recovered from a previous training session, LIT enables participants in our programs to train hard when the muscles are at their strongest.

> Since the greatest adaptations take place when the muscles have recovered from a previous training session, less intense training (LIT) enables participants to train hard when the muscles are at their strongest.

Youth in our strength-training programs typically perform an LIT session after more demanding training sessions. For example, if our high school athletes train with relatively heavy loads on Wednesday, they will perform an LIT session on the following workout. As a general guideline, during an LIT session participants will train at a reduced intensity while focusing on proper exercise technique. The LIT sessions may include several exercises for the major muscle groups as well as prehabilitation exercises for the lower-back and shoulder regions. That is, exercises that may be prescribed for the rehabilitation of an injury are performed beforehand as part of a preventive health measure. We have observed that LIT sessions that are sensibly incorporated into youth strength-training programs facilitate recovery and reduce the risk of injury while providing an excellent opportunity to reinforce key movement skills and optimize training adaptations (refer back to figure 13.1 on page 212).

In addition to varying the strength-training program, teachers and coaches need to pay just as much attention to what is done between training sessions as to what is done during training sessions. Strength training can place relatively high stress on the body, and therefore the importance of optimizing recovery needs to be reinforced regularly. This is particularly important for young athletes who are still growing, developing, and socializing with their friends. Youth coaches should realize that the "more is better" attitude is counterproductive and will likely result in injury, burnout, or poor performance. Along with healthy eating and adequate hydration (discussed in chapter 14), the following safe

and simple practices help youth recover from strength-training workouts:

- *Cool-down.* All workouts should end with a cool-down session that removes lactate and lessens the likelihood of muscle soreness. Calisthenics, light jogging, and static stretching have proven to be effective.
- *Contrast shower.* A postworkout contrast shower (alternating 30 seconds of warm water and 30 second of cold water for three or four cycles) can restore function and minimize inflammation after intense exercise.
- *Self-massage.* Foam rollers and massage sticks can minimize muscle stiffness and promote relaxation.

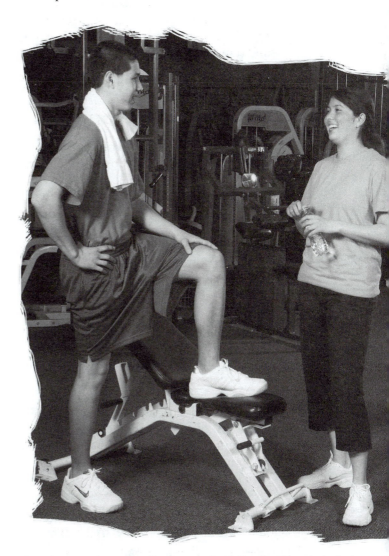

Socializing can have a positive impact on emotional and psychological well-being.

- *Adequate sleep.* Most youth need about 8 to 9 hours of sleep per night, and young athletes may need more than that. When appropriate, a power nap in the afternoon can help a child feel reenergized.
- *Music.* Listening to music can be a relaxing activity that can aid in the recovery process. Realize that the type of music used for maximizing recovery is a personal choice.
- *Socialization.* Youth should spend time with family, teammates, and people not involved in their sport. Social gatherings at school events or parties can have a positive impact on emotional and psychological well-being.
- *Visualization.* After practice and games, children should take a few quiet minutes to visualize the body recovering from the workout. Slow, deep breathing and thinking about getting stronger, feeling better, and removing soreness from your body will aid in the recovery process.

Long-Term Development

When working with school-age youth, remember that the long-term goal is to provide all participants with the skills, knowledge, and behaviors that will result in a lifetime of physical activity. While some boys and girls in our programs might become adult athletes, others will continue to participate in various types of physical activities as a lifestyle choice. In any case, instructors and coaches need to develop and enhance fundamental physical abilities in youth through regular participation in periodized programs that are consistent with each person's needs, goals, and abilities. This type of training enhances athleticism by providing youth with enough time to develop a variety of physical skills that require strength, power, endurance, flexibility, coordination, agility, and balance. In the long term, it is in the best interest of all youth to focus on enhancing fundamental fitness abilities rather than to focus on sport-specific performance.

> The long-term goal in working with youth is to provide all participants with the skills, knowledge, and behaviors that will result in a lifetime of physical activity.

Children and adolescents who participate only in sport programs will develop sport-specific skills and enhance their understanding of game strategy, but they will likely exhibit developmental gaps in their fundamental fitness abilities later in life. Although these young athletes may experience early success in sports, they also tend to suffer more injuries and seem to drop out of sports more often than youth who spend more time enhancing their overall athleticism during the developmental years. In many cases, the problems these athletes encounter as adults can be traced back to weak fundamentals during childhood and adolescence. Before young athletes face the pressure of competing in sports, they need to build a strong musculoskeletal foundation based on scientific principles.

In the long term, boys and girls who continue to enhance their fundamental abilities and knowledge of fitness will be better prepared to learn more advanced skills later in life. Professional athletes who make sport skills look easy likely spent many years working on fundamental fitness abilities during their youth. The results of their hard work are what we see on television. What we don't see is the physical conditioning that prepared their bodies for elite sport competition.

Summary

Periodization refers to the systematic variation of program variables for optimizing long-term training adaptations and reducing the likelihood of overtraining. In the long term, program variation with adequate rest and recovery between training sessions will allow children and adolescents to attain higher levels of muscular fitness because their bodies will be able to adapt to even greater demands. With a sensible use of the methods highlighted in this chapter, youth will optimize training adaptations and will be more likely to adhere to advanced training programs. Clearly, designing safe and effective youth strength-training programs involves an understanding of principles of strength training along with an appreciation for adequate rest and recovery between workouts. Knowledge gained from future studies will have a significant impact on how teachers and coaches prepare children and adolescents for a lifetime of strength training and sport participation.

14

EATING FOR STRENGTH AND PERFORMANCE

Now that you are ready to design a youth strength-training program, you might have some questions about proper nutrition and daily dietary requirements. You might have heard that strength training increases the need for protein, calcium, and other nutrients found in muscles and bones. Although this is true to some degree, it is neither necessary nor desirable to follow specialized diets or spend lots of money on food supplements. Generally, home-cooked meals that include a variety of grains, vegetables, fruits, and low-fat meat and dairy products are best from a nutritional perspective. Unfortunately, as society has become faster paced, home-cooked meals have become less common, and supermarket shelves have become well stocked with high-fat, high-sugar, and high-salt foods. It is not surprising that one problem many youth have is poor nutrition. Teachers and coaches need to recognize the importance of encouraging children and adolescents to eat nutritious foods to support growth, enhance health, and optimize fitness.

Weak nutrition can be defined as meals and snacks that are too high in saturated fat and sugar and too low in fiber and essential nutrients. The essential nutrients are protein (amino acids) for muscle development, carbohydrate for energy, fat for proper development and maintenance of the nervous system and all cells, minerals (especially calcium for bone development and potassium for regulating blood pressure and muscle contractions), vitamins, and water for all body functions. Many children and adolescents do not eat enough fruits and vegetables, and a growing number of youth do not meet dietary requirements for fiber. Current findings indicate that the average daily consumption of soft drinks continues to increase, whereas the consumption of milk, the largest source of bone-building calcium, has decreased over the past few years. Unfortunately, an overwhelming majority of food advertisements seen on television by children and adolescents are for products high in fat, sugar, and sodium.

Not only does weak nutrition limit gains in strength and increase the risk of fractures and anemia, but unhealthy eating contributes to obesity, diabetes, and heart disease. What's more, food preferences established early in life tend to carry over into adulthood. Children and adolescents need to eat a nutrient-dense diet that is rich in whole grains, fruits, vegetables, and low-fat meat and dairy products as well as essential vitamins, minerals, antioxidants, and fiber. In addition, youth need to limit the intake of saturated fat, trans fat, cholesterol, salt, and sugar. A nutrition discipline we call power eating restricts total fat intake to 25 percent of total calories (most of the fat comes from healthy polyunsaturated and monounsaturated sources) and increases nutrient-dense carbohydrate and protein to about 55 percent and 20 percent, respectively, of total caloric intake.

Basics of Healthy Eating

The new MyPyramid, developed by the United States Department of Agriculture, can help children and teens develop a personalized approach to healthy eating and physical activity. As illustrated in figure 14.1, MyPyramid includes several daily servings from the six food groups as well as essential vitamins and minerals to ensure ample energy. The varied widths of bands for the food groups suggest how much food should be chosen from each group. For example, the wider bands represent foods with little or no added fat or sugar (such as whole grains, vegetables, fruits, and milk) that should be selected more often, whereas the narrower bands represent foods containing more added sugar and fat. The person climbing the steps represents the importance of daily physical activity.

The MyPyramid Web site (www.mypyramid. gov) provides posters, food tracking worksheets, and sample menus that people can use in order to make smart food choices and get the most out of foods they eat. Since lack of knowledge about nutrition is not uncommon among school-age youth, children and adolescents can use interactive pages on the MyPyramid Web site to learn about healthy food choices and caloric needs from a reliable source. If additional information and guidance are needed, the American Dietetic Association (www.eatright.org) can help you find qualified nutrition professionals in your area who can provide personal assistance on a fee-for-service basis.

MyPyramid provides guidelines for healthy eating that apply to adults and youth. Because small children need less food, they should eat fewer servings than adults in each food category but maintain the same relative proportions. That

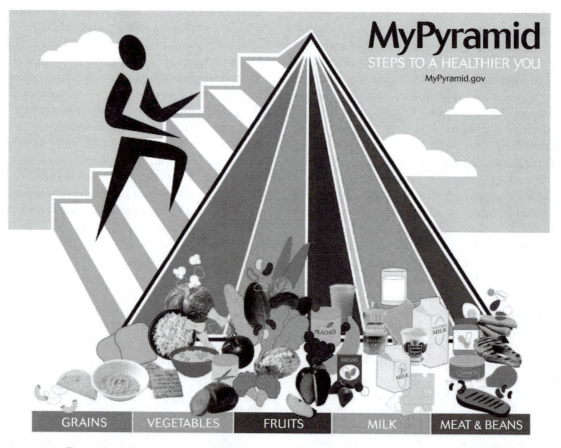

Figure 14.1 The MyPyramid graph.

U.S. Department of Agriculture and the U.S. Department of Health and Human Services or USDA and DHHS.

is, they should eat plenty of grains, vegetables, and fruit; moderate amounts of lean meat and low-fat dairy products; and low amounts of saturated fat, oil, and sweets. The following sections examine each food category more carefully.

> Because small children need less food, they should eat fewer servings than adults in each food category but maintain the same relative proportions. That is, they should eat plenty of grains, vegetables, and fruit; moderate amounts of lean meat and low-fat dairy products; and low amounts of saturated fat, oil, and sweets.

Grains

Grains include all kinds of foods made from wheat, oats, corn, rice, barley, and the like. Examples of grain foods are cereals, breads, pasta, pancakes, rice cakes, tortillas, bagels, muffins, corn bread, rice pudding, and chocolate cake. Obviously, some grain-based foods such as cakes, cookies, and pastries contain a lot of sugar and fat, and you should eat them sparingly. As mentioned, low-fat varieties of these foods are available in local supermarkets.

All grains are high in carbohydrate, and some grains or parts of grains, such as wheat germ, are also good sources of protein. Whole grains such as oatmeal, brown rice, and whole-wheat flour are typically rich in vitamins B_6, A, and E, as well as minerals such as zinc, copper, and iron. Whole grains are also good sources of soluble and insoluble fiber. Studies have shown that soluble fiber might help reduce blood cholesterol levels. Insoluble fiber helps with bowel regularity and may prevent gastrointestinal disorders. To determine whether a product contains whole grains, simply refer to the ingredients list. The first item should be labeled "whole" or "whole grain," such as whole wheat or whole cornmeal.

Refined grains, on the other hand, have been milled, which removes the bran and germ. While this process gives grains a finer texture and prolongs their shelf life, milling removes dietary fiber, iron, and many B vitamins. Examples of refined grain products are white bread and white rice. The number of recommended daily servings for whole grains is six; youth should eat at least three servings of *whole* grains every day. As a point of reference, one serving is 1 slice of bread, 1 cup (about 30 g) of ready-to-eat breakfast cereal, or half a cup (30 g) of cooked rice or pasta.

Vegetables

Like grains, vegetables are excellent sources of carbohydrate, vitamins, and fiber. Vegetables come in all sizes, shapes, colors, and nutritional characteristics and are low in calories. Orange vegetables are typically good sources of vitamin A and beta-carotene. This category includes carrots, sweet potatoes, and winter squash. Dark green vegetables are high in vitamins B_2 and folic acid. Some green vegetables are peas, beans, broccoli, asparagus, spinach, and lettuce. A light vinaigrette salad dressing accompanying any of these vegetables might be more appealing for a child. Red vegetables provide ample amounts of vitamin C. The best known vegetables in this category are tomatoes and red peppers. Other vegetables are essentially white, at least under the skin. These include cauliflower, summer squash, potatoes, and radishes, many of which are good sources of vitamin C.

In general, a cup (about 125 g) of raw or cooked vegetables or 2 cups (60 g) of raw leafy green vegetables count as one serving from the vegetable group. Youth should eat at least 2.5 cups (about 313 g) of vegetables every day. It is a good idea to eat some vegetables raw and to steam or microwave other vegetables for nutrient retention. In addition, fresh and frozen vegetables have more nutritional value and are lower in sodium than canned vegetables.

Fruit

Fruit, the counterpart to vegetables, is low in calories and has much variety and nutritional value. All fruit choices are high in carbohydrate and vitamins, and many provide excellent sources of fiber. A fruit's color often indicates the type of vitamin present. Table 14.1 presents examples of a variety of fruits in one-serving portions.

As you probably know, citrus fruits, such as oranges, grapefruit, and lemons, are loaded with vitamin C. Like orange-colored vegetables, orange-colored fruit, including cantaloupe, apricots, and papaya, are rich in vitamin A and

Table 14.1   Fruit: One Serving Size

2 tbsp raisins	1 pear	1/4 papaya
3 dates	3 apricots	1/2 mango
3 prunes	1/2 grapefruit	5 kumquats
1 cup grapes	1 cup pineapple	1 cup honeydew
1 apple	2 kiwi	1 cup strawberries
1 banana	1/2 pomegranate	1 cup watermelon
1 peach	1/4 cantaloupe	

beta-carotene. Both green fruit, such as honeydew melon and kiwi, and red fruit, such as strawberries and cherries, are high in vitamin C. Yellow fruit includes peaches, mangos, and pineapples, all of which are good sources of vitamin C. Fruit that is white, at least on the inside, includes apples, pears, and bananas, all of which are high in potassium.

Dried fruits are nutrient dense, and the natural sweetness makes them healthy substitutes for high-fat snacks such as candy bars. Raisins, dates, figs, and prunes are all superb energy sources, and prunes are the single best source of dietary fiber. Note that one serving varies considerably, depending on the type of fruit. For example, 1 cup of fresh fruit and half a cup of the dried version of that same fruit are equal in calories and vitamins. The difference is water content. Fresh fruit contains lots of water, whereas dried fruit is a high-density carbohydrate. If children prefer fruit in liquid form, 8 ounces (about 240 ml) of 100 percent fruit juice equals one serving but has less fiber than whole fruit. In any case, consider the calorie content of these beverages when encouraging children to eat at least 2 cups of fruit every day.

Milk Products

MyPyramid recommends three servings of dairy products, including low-fat or nonfat milk, yogurt, and cheese, every day for youth older than eight years; two servings are recommended for children two to eight years. Eight ounces (about 227 g) of milk or yogurt, 1.5 ounces (about 45 g) of natural cheese, or 2 ounces (60 g) of processed cheese count as one serving from the milk group. These foods are excellent sources of protein and calcium. Because whole-milk products are high in fat, be selective at the dairy case. For example, low-fat milk and nonfat yogurt offer heart-healthy alternatives to high-fat dairy selections. Although there are many other sources of dietary calcium, children often have difficulty obtaining sufficient calcium unless they regularly consume products in the milk group. If a child has problems digesting milk (lactose intolerance), choose lactose-free products and try to regularly provide other foods that are high in calcium, such as dark green leafy greens, beans, and legumes. Also, a variety of calcium-fortified foods, such as orange juice, are now available at most supermarkets.

Meat and Beans

This category includes meat, poultry, fish, eggs, beans (dried beans, chickpeas, lentils, and split peas), nuts, and seeds. All these foods are good sources of protein, although some also contain significant amounts of fat. MyPyramid recommends eating 5.5 servings of food from this group every day. One ounce of meat, poultry, or fish; one egg; one tablespoon of peanut butter; a quarter cup (45 g) of cooked dried beans; or half an ounce (15 g) of nuts or seeds count as one serving from the meat and bean category. Table 14.2 presents sample foods in the meat category according to their fat content. Note that how you prepare the food has a lot to do with how much fat it contains. Obviously, baking, broiling, or grilling meat is a better choice than frying.

Although there are differences in fat content, the amount of protein found in one serving is somewhat consistent throughout the various types of food in this category. As you can see from

Table 14.2   Fat Content of Meat, Fish, Poultry, and Eggs

Low fat	Medium fat	High fat
All fish (not fried)	Chicken with skin	Beef ribs
Egg whites	Turkey with skin	Pork ribs
Chicken without skin	Roast beef	Corned beef
Turkey without skin	Roast pork	Sausage
Venison	Roast lamb	Lunch meat
Rabbit	Veal cutlet	Ground pork
Top round	Ground beef	Hot dogs
Eye of round	Steak	Fried chicken
Sirloin		
Flank steak		

Table 14.3   Meat and Beans: Equivalent Portion Sizes

3 oz fish (salmon, tuna)	3 tbsp peanut butter
3 oz poultry (chicken, turkey)	0.75 cup cooked dried beans
3 oz meat (beef, poultry, lamb, etc.)	1.5 oz nuts or seeds
3 eggs	0.75 cup tofu

table 14.3, 3 ounces of meat, poultry, and fish (about the size of a deck of cards) have roughly the same amount of protein as 0.75 cup of cooked dried beans and 1.5 ounces of nuts and seeds. While most meat and poultry choices should be lean or low fat, realize that fish such as salmon, tuna, and trout contain healthy oils and therefore should be eaten more often. On the whole, it is beneficial to make varied choices from this food group, including nuts and seeds (especially almonds and sunflower seeds), which are good sources of vitamin E and essential fatty acids. Just remember to keep track of the serving size because nuts and seeds are calorie dense.

Oil

The smallest band of MyPyramid is the oil group, which refers to fat that is liquid at room temperature. Foods that are mainly oil, such as mayonnaise and certain salad dressings, should be consumed sparingly. Although all types of fat contain 9 calories per gram, some types of fat are more desirable than others from a health perspective. For example, consuming saturated fat (such as that found in butter and shortening) puts a person at higher risk for developing heart disease than eating monounsaturated fat (such as that found in olive oil and canola oil) and polyunsaturated fat (such as that found in corn oil). See table 14.4 to determine serving equivalents for foods in the oil group.

Young children are especially vulnerable to consumption of high-fat food when you consider that many fast-food restaurants offer special incentives. Prepackaged meals typically include hamburgers, cheeseburgers, or batter-dipped chicken tenders with french fries and a choice of drink. The main attraction, however, is that these meals come with a special toy in the bag, usually depicting a character from the most recent children's animated films. Children not only want

Table 14.4   Oil: One Serving Size

1 tsp butter	1 tbsp cream cheese
1 tsp margarine	2 tbsp light cream cheese
1 tbsp diet margarine	2 tbsp sour cream
1 tsp mayonnaise	4 tbsp light sour cream
1 tbsp diet mayonnaise	1 tbsp salad dressing
1 tsp oil	2 tbsp diet salad dressing

the toy, but they also want to collect all the toys featured in the collection, which lures them into a cycle of fast-food selections. What a difference it would make in our children's lives if the pre-packaged meal with a toy offered foods low in fat and high in nutrients rather than the opposite.

Children's Nutritional Needs

Although MyPyramid presents a healthy and personalized eating pattern, many youth follow a completely opposite nutritional lifestyle. It is not unusual for teens and preteens to eat far more candy bars, corn chips, french fries, cheese-burgers, and ice cream (all of which are 50 to 80 percent fat) than apples, oranges, bananas, salads, cooked vegetables, rice, whole grains, fish, chicken, low-fat milk, and yogurt. Of course, the latter foods are low in fat and high in nutrients, making them much better selections. However, motivating youth to want to follow our power eating plan is a key to developing a healthier lifestyle for the child. You can do this in the following ways.

First, encourage healthy eating patterns early. While the child is young, teach him or her to enjoy trying new fruits such as seedless clementines or papayas. If a child sees an adult eating something new, and if it looks good, the child will naturally be curious. To go one step further, when a child sees something new and does not have the alternative choice of a high-fat snack, he or she will naturally opt for what is available. Another idea is to make certain snacks a tradition. For families, if Friday night is family time, be sure to have staples on hand, such as raw baby carrots and fat-free ranch dressing. Carrots are naturally

sweet and children love them. Another popular idea is sliced apples with cinnamon.

Role modeling plays an important part in developing healthy eating habits in children. Adults tend to eat the snacks most readily available in the household and at social events, and children will follow suit. If a child sees an adult eating a bag of potato chips, the child is going to reach for the same thing. If an adult routinely enjoys high-sugar or high-fat snacks, how can that adult say no when the child asks for the same? When choosing store-bought snacks, opt for the ones that are low in saturated fat. This does not mean that children (and adults) should not enjoy occasional pizzas or cookies with milk, but you should balance foods high in saturated fat with several selections from the vegetable, fruit, and grain categories daily. In any case, special care must be taken when planning healthy meals and snacks for youth so that they consume a variety of nutrient-dense foods and beverages that are essential for normal growth and development.

> Role modeling plays an important part in developing healthy eating habits in children. If a child sees an adult eating a bag of potato chips, the child is going to reach for the same thing.

Protein Requirements

While sufficient protein is essential for growth and repair, the body does not use extra protein if the protein supply is currently sufficient. Most children and adolescents eat more than enough protein from food to satisfy all their muscle-building requirements. The body simply puts the excess protein into storage after the liver converts it to fat. Moreover, too much protein can increase the risk of dehydration and might cause calcium loss from bones.

How much protein is necessary for youth who participate in strength-training programs? Generally, 1 gram of protein for every kilogram (about 2 pounds) of body weight is recommended for meeting the metabolic needs and muscle-building requirements of most children and teens. While some young athletes may need slightly more protein, the little scientific information that is available on this topic makes it difficult to make specific recommendations. For example, a boy or girl who weighs 100 pounds (45 kg) should eat at least 50 grams of protein a day. Because an ounce (30 g) of meat (e.g., fish, chicken, turkey, lean beef) contains about 7 grams of protein, 8 ounces of meat should fulfill the daily protein requirement. Likewise, 1 cup (240 ml) of low-fat dairy products (e.g., milk, yogurt, cottage cheese) contains about 8 grams of protein. Therefore, three servings of low-fat dairy foods provide about half the daily need for protein. Because most youth typically consume at least this much meat and milk as well as other protein-containing foods daily, their muscles should be well supplied with protein and highly responsive to strength exercise.

Some youth follow a vegetarian diet, which can be a very healthy way to eat with proper planning. A vegan (total vegetarian) diet includes only food from plants, but other vegetarian eating plans, such as the ovolactovegetarian diet, are less restrictive and include dairy and egg products but no red meat. In any case, children and teens who follow a vegetarian diet need to be sure they make healthy food choices so that they do not miss out on important nutrients, including protein, iron, and vitamin B_{12}. Since a teenager's perception of a vegetarian meal (e.g., french fries and soda) might not be consistent with a healthy eating plan, consultation with a qualified nutrition professional can help in planning and monitoring a vegetarian diet that includes nutritious food choices.

Vitamins and Minerals

Many people believe that humans do not obtain enough vitamins and minerals from daily meals. But this is true only if people do not eat a variety of foods as recommended in MyPyramid. Youth

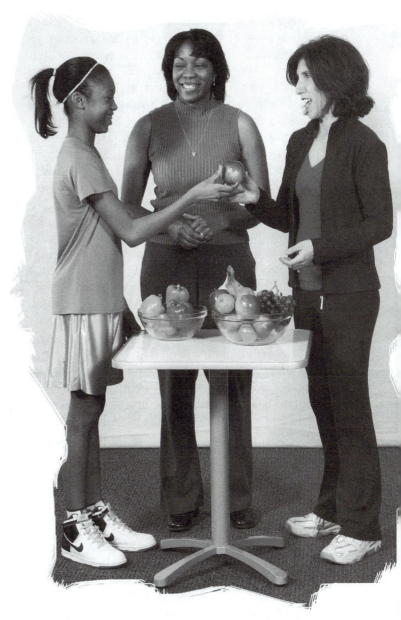

Educate children and their parents about healthy food choices.

and adults who consume several daily servings of grains, vegetables, and fruit and a few servings of meat and milk should not lack any essential vitamins or minerals.

Of course, children who do not eat regular or varied meals may risk vitamin or mineral deficiency. Although children can remedy this problem by taking daily vitamin and mineral supplements, it is preferable to obtain nutrients from food. In addition to providing protein, carbohydrate, fat, vitamins, and minerals, foods supply bulk and fiber necessary for desirable digestion and elimination.

For developing strong bones, it is important to realize that vitamin D is just as important as calcium. Although fortified milk is an excellent source of Vitamin D, dairy products made from milk, such as cheese, yogurt, and ice cream, are generally not fortified with vitamin D. Fortified cereals and selected types of fish, including salmon, mackerel, and sardines, are good food sources of vitamin D. Interestingly, vitamin D can also be made by the skin when it is exposed to sunlight. About 10 to 15 minutes of sun exposure without sunscreen several times per week is usually sufficient in providing adequate vitamin D.

Recently there has been considerable emphasis on antioxidant vitamins, especially vitamins A, C, and E. Fortunately, it is not difficult to get these vitamins through healthy eating habits. For example, vitamin C is prevalent in citrus fruits and juices, tomatoes, potatoes, peppers, strawberries, melons, and many other fruits and vegetables. Vitamin A is found in most orange foods, such as cantaloupe, carrots, squash, sweet potatoes, and apricots. The best sources of vitamin E are wheat germ and fish, but you can also it is also present in sweet potatoes, almonds, and sunflower seeds.

Carbohydrate

Eating appropriate energy-releasing foods before and after strength workouts can enhance the training effort and recovery processes. Carbohydrate is the real power food that serves as the primary energy source for strength exercise. Although all types of carbohydrate (grains, fruits, and vegetables) supplies fuel for physical activity, some release energy slowly and others release energy quickly. Carbohydrate that breaks down slowly has a low glycemic index, and we recommend them before working out because they provide sustained energy. Carbohydrate that breaks down quickly has a high glycemic index because it enters the bloodstream fast and rapidly replenishes energy stores after exercising.

Before training, children should eat foods that have a low glycemic index, including carrots, apples, pears, chocolate milk, low-fat fruit yogurt, dried apricots, bananas, and whole milk. After training, children should eat foods that have a high glycemic index, including cornflakes, rice cakes, vanilla wafers, graham crackers, honey, bagels, and raisins.

Hydration

In addition to healthy food choices, one of the most important components of power eating is adequate hydration, so active youth should drink at least eight glasses of water (or healthy caffeine-free alternatives such as fruit juices or low-fat milk) every day. Keep in mind that muscle is over 75 percent water, and a decrease in body weight of only 1 percent through exercise-induced sweating negatively affects performance. Since levels of dehydration of 2 to 3 percent body weight are not uncommon in young athletes, every effort should be made to ensure that boys and girls arrive to every workout fully hydrated and drink fluid before, during, and after the exercise session. Here is a general rule: Urine will be pale yellow in color (like lemonade) when fluid levels are adequate, and urine will be dark gold in color (like apple juice) when a person is dehydrated.

> One of the most important components of power eating is adequate hydration, so active youth should drink at least eight glasses of water (or healthy caffeine-free alternatives) every day.

During a workout, youth should stay hydrated by drinking cool beverages every 15 to 20 minutes. Since children do not tolerate heat as well as older athletes, it is particularly important to ensure adequate fluid intake when exercising in a hot environment. Although water is best for activities lasting less than one hour, some boys and girls find the taste of sport drinks more palatable and therefore are more likely to drink regularly and avoid voluntary dehydration. We encourage youth to take a water bottle to school and drink between classes and during breaks so that they are hydrated for afterschool fitness activities.

Snack Foods

We often ask children to avoid snacks between meals so that they will have a good appetite for healthy foods at breakfast, lunch, and dinner. Although this is good advice, active boys and girls can benefit from preworkout and postworkout snacks. These energy-replacement selections should be small, nutritious, and accompanied with fluids. We encourage participants in our youth strength-training classes to take advantage of the "golden hour" after exercise by consuming a snack or beverage containing carbohydrate and protein. This will quickly refuel carbohydrate stores and result in a faster buildup of muscle proteins.

Here are some healthy snacking ideas children enjoy:

- 100 percent apple juice, orange juice, or vegetable juice
- Banana and low-fat milk
- Raisins and nuts
- Sliced apples with cinnamon
- Celery with a thin layer of peanut butter
- Carrot sticks with nonfat ranch dressing
- Low-fat yogurt or cottage cheese
- Seedless grapes or clementines

Children who crave sweet foods might want to substitute dried fruit (e.g., raisins, dates, figs, prunes, apricots) for candy and pastries. Dried fruit provides similar sweetness but contains almost no fat, making it a much healthier snack food than candy and pastries. Children who prefer high-sugar cereals might enjoy honey nut varieties.

Youth who like to munch on chips can eat unsalted nuts or seeds (e.g., almonds, pecans, cashews, peanuts, sunflower seeds) as crunchy alternatives. Although nuts and seeds are high in oil, they contain many valuable nutrients and are healthier than foods high in saturated fat.

Children who crave sweet foods might want to substitute dried fruit (e.g., raisins, dates, figs, prunes, apricots) for candy and pastries.

Summary

There are many benefits of establishing healthy eating patterns at an early age. First, proper nutrition provides a child with the necessary energy, nutrients, and building blocks to maintain an active lifestyle. Second, encouraging positive food choices can help a child continue similar behaviors into adulthood. Finally, although the effects of eating high-fat foods might not be evident for many years, food choices made in childhood have just as much impact on overall health as those made in adult life. Therefore it is important to work with parents, school administrators, and health care providers to replace high-fat, low-nutrient fast foods with alternatives that benefit children's health and fitness. You can do this by educating through example and by providing healthy options that maximize muscle development and energy production, minimize fat accumulation, and truly appeal to children and adolescents. As a result, youth will have the knowledge, energy, enthusiasm, and equilibrium they need for a happy and healthy future in fitness.

SAMPLE WORKOUT LOG

Name: Rita Sanchez
Age: 12

Date		9/18	9/21									
	Settings	\multicolumn{11}{c}{**Weights\reps**}									
Warm-up		✓	✓									
Leg press	5	10 / 80	12 / 80									
Leg extension	4	10 / 20	11 / 20									
Leg curl	4	10 / 10	11 / 10									
Chest press	2	10 / 8	12 / 8									
Seated row	3	10 / 15	12 / 15									
Lateral raise		10 / 3	12 / 3									
Triceps extension	3	10 / 3	12 / 3									
Biceps curl	3	10 / 3	12 / 3									
Medicine ball lower-back pull		10 / 2	11 / 2									
Medicine ball curl-up		10 / 2	12 / 2									
Medicine ball twist		10 / 2	12 / 2									
Cool-down stretches		✓	✓									

SUGGESTED READINGS

American Academy of Pediatrics. 2008. Strength training by children and adolescents. *Pediatrics,* 121: 835-840.

American College of Sports Medicine. 2007. *ACSM's guidelines for exercise testing and prescription.* 7th ed. Baltimore: Lippincott, Williams & Wilkins.

American Council on Exercise. 2009. *ACEs advanced health & fitness specialist manual.* C. Bryant & D. Green (Eds.). Monterey, CA: Healthy Learning.

Annesi, J., Westcott, W., Faigenbaum, A., & Unruh, J. 2005. Effects of a 12-week physical activity protocol delivered by YMCA after-school counselors on fitness and self-efficacy changes in 5-12-year-old boys and girls. *Research Quarterly for Exercise and Sport,* 76: 468-476.

Behm, D., Faigenbaum, A., Falk, B., & Klentrou, P. 2008. Canadian Society for Exercise Physiology position paper: Resistance training in children and adolescents. *Journal of Applied Physiology Nutrition Metabolism,* 33: 547-561.

Benson, A., Torade, M., & Fiatarone, M. 2008. Effects of resistance training on metabolic fitness in children and adolescents. *Obesity Reviews,* 9: 43-66.

British Association of Exercise and Sport Sciences. 2004. BASES position statement on guidelines for resistance exercise in young people. *Journal of Sports Sciences,* 22: 383-390.

Chu, D., Faigenbaum, A., & Falkel, J. 2006. *Progressive plyometrics for kids.* Monterey, CA: Healthy Learning.

Cooper Institute for Aerobics Research. 1999. *Fitness-gram test administration manual.* 2nd ed. Champaign, IL: Human Kinetics.

Faigenbaum, A. 2007. Resistance training for children and adolescents: Are there health outcomes? *American Journal of Lifestyle Medicine,* 1: 190-200.

Faigenbaum, A., Farrell, A., Radler, T., Zbojovsky, D., Chu, D., Ratamess, N., Kang, J., & Hoffman, J. 2009. "Plyo Play": A novel program of short bouts of moderate and high intensity exercise improves physical fitness in elementary school children. *The Physical Educator,* 66: 37-44.

Faigenbaum, A., Kang, J., McFarland, J., Bloom, J., Magnatta, J.. Ratamess, N., & Hoffman, J. 2006. Acute effects of different warm-up protocols on anaerobic performance in teenage athletes. *Pediatric Exercise Science,* 17: 64-75.

Faigenbaum, A., Kraemer, W., Blimkie, C., Jeffreys, I., Micheli, L., Nitka, M., & Rowland, T. In press. Youth resistance training: Updated position statement paper from the National Strength and Conditioning Association. *Journal of Strength & Conditioning Research.*

Faigenbaum, A., & McFarland, J. 2007. Guidelines for implementing a dynamic warm-up for physical education. *Journal of Physical Education, Recreation and Dance,* 78: 25-28.

Faigenbaum, A., McFarland, J., Johnson, L., Kang, J., Bloom, J., Ratamess, N., & Hoffman, J. 2007. Preliminary evaluation of an after-school resistance training program. *Perceptual Motor Skills,* 104: 407-415.

Faigenbaum, A., McFarland, J., Keiper, F., Tevlin, W., Kang, J., Ratamess, N., & Hoffman J. 2007. Effects of a short term plyometric and resistance training program on fitness performance in boys age 12 to 15 years. *Journal of Sports Science and Medicine,* 6: 519-525.

Faigenbaum, A., McFarland, J., Schwerdtman, J., Ratamess, N., Kang, N., & Hoffman, J. 2006. Dynamic warm-up protocols, with and without a weighted vest, and fitness performance in high school female athletes. *Journal of Athletic Training,* 41: 357-363.

Faigenbaum, A., & Mediate, P. 2006. The effects of medicine ball training on physical fitness in high school physical education students, *The Physical Educator,* 63: 160-167.

Faigenbaum, A., Milliken, L., Cloutier, C., & Westcott, W. 2004. Perceived exertion during resistance exercise in children. *Perceptual Motor Skills,* 98: 627-637.

Faigenbaum, A. Milliken, L., LaRosa Loud, R., Burak, B., Doherty, C. & Westcott, W. 2002. Comparison of 1 day and 2 days per week of strength training in children. *Research Quarterly for Exercise and Sport,* 73: 416-424.

Faigenbaum, A., Milliken, L., & Westcott, W. 2003. Maximal strength testing in children. *Journal of Strength and Conditioning Research,* 17: 162-166.

Faigenbaum, A., Ratamess, N., McFarland, J., Kaczmarek, J., Coraggio, M., Kang, J., & Hoffman, J. 2008. Effect of rest interval length on bench press performance in boys, teens and men. *Pediatric Exercise Science*, 20: 457-469.

Faigenbaum, A., & Westcott, W. 2001. *Youth fitness.* San Diego: American Council on Exercise.

Faigenbaum, A., & Westcott, W. *Youth strength training.* 2005. San Diego: American Council on Exercise.

Faigenbaum, A., & Westcott, W. 2007. Resistance training for obese children and adolescents. *President's Council on Physical Fitness and Sports Research Digest*, 8: 1-8.

Faigenbaum, A., Westcott, W., Larosa Loud, R., & Long, C. 1999. The effects of different resistance training protocols on muscular strength and endurance development in children. *Pediatrics*, 104: e5.

Faigenbaum, A., Westcott, W., Micheli, L., Outerbridge, A., Long, C., LaRosa Loud, R., & Zaichkowsky, L. 1996. The effects of strength training and detraining on children. *Journal of Strength and Conditioning Research*, 10: 109-114.

Faigenbaum, A., Zaichkowsky, L., Westcott, W., Micheli, L., and Fehlandt, A. 1993. The effects of a twice per week strength training program on children. *Pediatric Exercise Science*, 5: 339-346.

Hamill, B. Relative safety of weight lifting and weight training. 1994. *Journal of Strength & Conditioning Research*, 8: 53-57.

Hebestreit, H., & Bar-Or, O. (Eds.). 2008. *The young athlete.* Malden, MA: Blackwell.

Hoffman, J. 2006. *Norms for health, fitness, and performance.* Champaign IL: Human Kinetics.

Jeffreys, I. 2008. *Coaches guide to enhancing recovery in athletes: A multidimensional approach to developing the performance lifestyle.* Monterey, CA: Healthy Learning.

Malina, R. 2006. Weight training in youth-growth, maturation and safety: an evidenced based review. *Clinical Journal of Sport Medicine*, 16:478-487.

Malina, R., Bouchard, C., & Bar-Or, O. 2004. *Growth, maturation, and physical activity.* 2nd ed. Champaign, IL: Human Kinetics.

Mediate, P., & Faigenbaum, A. 2007. *Medicine ball for all kids.* Monterey, CA: Healthy Learning.

Micheli, L., Glassman, R., & Klein, M. 2000. The prevention of sports injuries in youth. *Clinical Sports Medicine*, 19: 821-834.

Micheli, L., & Purcell, L. 2007. *The adolescent athlete: A practical approach.* New York: Springer.

Milliken, L., Faigenbaum, A., LaRosa Loud, R., & Westcott, W. 2008. Correlates of upper and lower body muscular strength in children. *Journal of Strength & Conditioning Research*, 22: 1-8.

Mountjoy, M., Armstrong, N., Bizzini, L., Blimkie, C., Evans, J., Gerrard, D., Hangen, J., Knoll, K., Micheli, L., Sangenis, P., & Van Mechelen, W. 2008. IOC consensus statement: Training the elite young athlete. *Clinical Journal of Sport Medicine*, 18: 122-123.

National Association for Sport and Physical Education. 2005. *Physical education for lifelong fitness.* 2nd ed. Champaign, IL: Human Kinetics.

National Strength and Conditioning Association. 2008. *Essentials of strength training and conditioning.* 3rd ed. T. Baechle & R. Earle (Eds.). Champaign, IL: Human Kinetics.

Ortega, F., Ruiz, J., Castillo, M., & Sjostrom, M. 2008. Physical fitness in childhood and adolescence: a powerful marker of health. *International Journal of Obesity*, 32: 1-11.

Roberts, S., Ciapponi, T., & Lytle, R. 2008. *Strength training for children and adolescents.* Reston, VA: National Association for Sports and Physical Education.

Rowland, T. 2005. *Children's exercise physiology.* 2nd ed. Champaign, IL: Human Kinetics.

Strong, W., Malina, R., Blimkie, C., Daniels, S., Dishman, R., Gutin, B., Hergenroeder, A., Must, A., Nixon, P., Pivarnik, J., Rowland, T., Trost, S., & Trudeau, F. 2005. Evidence based physical activity for school-age youth. *Journal of Pediatrics*, 146: 732-737.

Vaughn, J., & Micheli, L. 2008. Strength training recommendations for the young athlete. *Physical Medicine and Rehabilitation Clinics of North America*, 19: 235-245.

Westcott, W. 1979. Female response to weight lifting. *Journal of Physical Education*, 77: 31-33.

Westcott, W., Tolken, J., & Wessner, B. 1995. School-based conditioning programs for physically unfit children. *Strength and Conditioning Journal*, 17: 5-9.

INDEX

Note: The italicized *f* and *t* following page numbers refer to figures and tables, respectively.

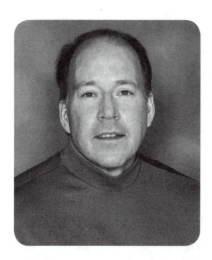

Avery D. Faigenbaum, EdD, CSCS, is a professor in the department of health and exercise science at the College of New Jersey. Dr. Faigenbaum is a leading researcher and practitioner in pediatric exercise science, with nearly 20 years of experience in working with children and adolescents. He has authored more than 100 scientific articles, 20 book chapters, and 7 books related to youth fitness and conditioning. In addition, Dr. Faigenbaum has lectured nationally and internationally to health and fitness organizations and has developed youth fitness programs for YMCAs, recreation centers, physical education classes, and after-school sport programs.

Dr. Faigenbaum is a fellow of the American College of Sports Medicine and of the National Strength and Conditioning Association. He is also a member of the International Scientific Advisory Committee and was a member of the Massachusetts Governor's Council on Physical Fitness and Sports for 7 years.

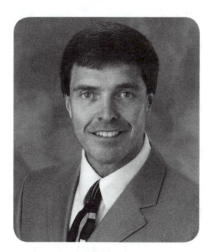

Wayne L. Westcott, PhD, CSCS, is a fitness research director at the South Shore YMCA and instructor of exercise science at Quincy College, both in Quincy, Massachusetts. He has served as a strength-training consultant for Nautilus, the United States Navy, the American Council on Exercise, the President's Council on Physical Fitness and Sports, and the YMCA of the USA. He has also been an editorial advisor for many publications, including *Physician and Sportsmedicine, Fitness Management, On-Site Fitness, Prevention, Shape,* and *Men's Health.* He has authored or coauthored 23 books on strength training worldwide and has helped numerous colleges, schools, YMCAs, and fitness centers develop youth strength-training programs.

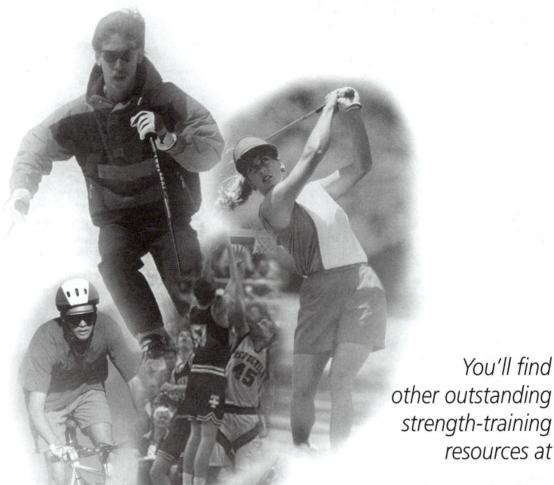